Non-alcoholic Fatty Liver Disease - New Insight and Glance Into Disease Pathogenesis

Edited by Ju-Seop Kang

Published in London, United Kingdom

Non-alcoholic Fatty Liver Disease - New Insight and Glance Into Disease Pathogenesis
http://dx.doi.org/10.5772/intechopen.100998
Edited by Ju-Seop Kang

Contributors
Li Yang, Shuo Zhang, Bing Ji, Changqing Yang, Georgios Sfikas, Ioannis Valsamidis, Ibrahim Kalle Kwaifa, Abdullahi S. Mainasara, Muhammad Lawal Jidda, Amrina Mohammad Amin, Garba Abdullahi Abdullahi, Faruk Ladan, Maryam Danyaro, Yuki Hamada, Eiichi Hirano, Shadi Hamoud, Bangyan L. Stiles, Brittney Hua, Aditi A. Datta, Chenxi Xu, Chien-yu Chen, Ielyzaveta Slarve

First published in London, United Kingdom, 2023 by IntechOpen
IntechOpen is the global imprint of INTECHOPEN LIMITED, registered in England and Wales, registration number: 11086078, 5 Princes Gate Court, London, SW7 2QJ, United Kingdom

British Library Cataloguing-in-Publication Data
A catalogue record for this book is available from the British Library

Additional hard and PDF copies can be obtained from orders@intechopen.com

Non-alcoholic Fatty Liver Disease - New Insight and Glance Into Disease Pathogenesis
Edited by Ju-Seop Kang
p. cm.
Print ISBN 978-1-83968-090-8
Online ISBN 978-1-83968-091-5
eBook (PDF) ISBN 978-1-83968-102-8

Meet the editor

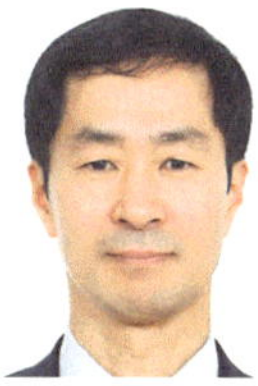

Prof. Ju-Seop Kang received his medical degree from Hanyang University College of Medicine, South Korea. He is currently a professor and director of the Department of Pharmacology and Clinical Pharmacology at the same university. He is also on the committee for the Department of Research Integrity at Hanyang University and a member of the appraisal committee of the Korea Medical Dispute Mediation and Arbitration Agency of the Ministry of Health and Welfare. He has published more than 100 papers in peer-reviewed international journals and 10 book chapters. He is a reviewer for five international journals and on the editorial board of several others.

Contents

Preface

Non-alcoholic fatty liver disease (NAFLD) is the leading primary cause of chronic liver disease in both children and adults worldwide. Global prevalence is estimated at 25% and accounts for the most common etiology of abnormal liver function tests in Western countries. NAFLD is a clinical-histopathologic entity with histologic features that resemble alcohol-induced liver injury, but by definition it occurs in patients with little or no history of alcohol consumption. It encompasses a histologic spectrum that ranges from fat accumulation in hepatocytes without concomitant inflammation or fibrosis (simple hepatic steatosis) to hepatic steatosis with a necroinflammatory component (steatohepatitis) that may or may not have associated fibrosis. The latter condition, referred to as nonalcoholic steatohepatitis (NASH), may progress to cirrhosis in up to 20% of patients. NASH is now recognized to be a leading cause of cryptogenic cirrhosis.

The pathogenesis of NAFLD has not been fully elucidated. The most widely supported theory implicates insulin resistance as the key mechanism leading to hepatic steatosis, and perhaps also to steatohepatitis. Others have proposed that a "second hit," or additional oxidative injury, is required to manifest the necroinflammatory component of steatohepatitis. Hepatic iron, gut hormones, antioxidant deficiencies, and intestinal bacteria have all been implicated in the pathogenesis of NAFLD.

This book includes contributions from global experts that present and discusses the most current results and theory for the pathogenesis of NAFLD. In addition to the knowledge shared, the authors provide their personal experimental experience, making this book an extremely useful tool for researchers in this field. Chapters discuss hepatic iron metabolism, the role of heparanase, ERR regulation, lipid homeostasis, therapeutic approaches, and HDL as a molecular modifier in the pathogenesis of NAFLD.

Ju-Seop Kang MD, Ph.D.
Professor of Pharmacology and Clinical Pharmacology,
College of Medicine,
Hanyang University,
Seoul, South Korea

Section 1

Basic Concept and Molecular Aspect in the Development of NAFLD/NASH

Chapter 1

Non-Alcoholic Fatty Liver Disease: Pathogenesis and the Significance of High-Density Lipoprotein as a Molecular Modifier

Ibrahim Kalle Kwaifa, Abdullahi S. Mainasara, Muhammad Lawal Jidda, Amrina Mohammad Amin, Garba Abdullahi, Faruku Ladan and Maryam Danyaro

Abstract

The pathophysiology of non-alcoholic fatty liver disease (NAFLD) can be identified by modifications in lifestyle, diet and inflammation, all of which have significant implications for the severity of the clinicopathologic outcome of the disease. Prolonged accumulation of hepatic lipid may result in hepatic dysfunction, inflammation and advanced forms of NAFLD. NAFLD describes the presence of hepatic steatosis in the absence of alcohol use and other causes of liver disease. It covers a broad spectrum of hepatic histopathological alterations, from a non-inflammatory intracellular accumulation of fat to non-alcoholic steatohepatitis (NASH), which may progress to hepatic fibrosis, cirrhosis, or hepatocellular carcinoma (HCC). Previous evidence has shown that NAFLD is associated with a range of metabolic syndromes, including obesity, hyperlipidaemia, insulin resistance and diabetes. Hepatic fibrosis and cirrhosis are more common in people with NAFLD, which is partly associated with hyperlipidaemia and low high-density lipoprotein-cholesterol (HDL-C) levels. The ability of HDL to facilitate cholesterol efflux, as determined by cholesterol efflux capacity (CEC), has been linked to its hepatoprotective functions in the body. Findings have demonstrated that NAFLD patients have suppressed HDL CEC. This chapter summarizes the molecular mechanisms and pathogenesis involved in NAFLD. The role of HDL as a molecular modulator of NAFLD, clinical implications and the therapeutic targets to prevent NAFLD have also been discussed.

Keywords: high-density lipoprotein, non-alcoholic fatty liver disease, pathogenesis and therapeutic targets

1. Introduction

Non-alcoholic fatty liver disease is defined as a broad spectrum of hepatic histopathological changes, from a non-inflammatory intracellular accumulation of lipid to

NASH, which can develop into hepatic fibrosis, cirrhosis, or HCC [1]. NAFLD is the excessive hepatic deposition of neutral lipids, initiated by an imbalance between lipid availability and clearance. Hepatic lipid accumulation in NAFLD is caused by changes in intracellular cholesterol transport and imbalanced cellular cholesterol homeostasis, characterized by the activations of cholesterol biosynthetic pathways. Enhanced cholesterol de-esterification, modulations of bile acid synthetic pathways and cholesterol export [2]. Through the activation of intracellular signaling pathways in Kupffer cells (KCs), hepatic Stellate cells (HSCs), and hepatocytes, the hepatic lipids accumulation causes liver damage, inflammation and fibrogenesis. Additionally, the mitochondrial dysfunction in the liver may cause an increase in the formation of reactive oxygen species (ROS), which could in turn causes endoplasmic reticulum (ER) stress and death by triggering the unfolded protein response [2]. These actions result in a vicious cycle that supports the progress of steatosis, liver damage and hepatocyte death, which may eventually result in disease progression. Triglycerides (TG) and HDL-C frequently undergo distinctive alterations in atherogenic dyslipidaemia, which is intimately associated with NAFLD. Indeed, atherogenic dyslipidaemia is closely linked to NAFLD, attributed to modifications in TG and HDL-C, hence, constant monitoring of atherosclerotic lipids is essential to evaluate the risk of NAFLD [1, 3, 4].

The incidence of NAFLD is currently around 25% worldwide, with a significant regional variation in the Middle East (32%), South America (31%) as well as the United States (24.1%) and Africa (14%). The prevalence also varies with metabolic disorders, which indicated that approximately 90% of obese individuals, 65% of overweight people, and up to 70% of diabetes mellitus (DM) patients have NAFLD. NAFLD has also been investigated in most ethnic groups but with a lower prevalence in African Americans compared with European-Americans and Hispanics [2, 5]. HDL-C has been considered to modulate NAFLD through several pathways that promote cholesterol efflux in the system, including the reverse cholesterol transport pathway [2, 5], however, essential information to fully understand the impact of HDL-C in NAFLD are limited. In this review, progress on the existing knowledge of the dysregulated cholesterol homeostasis in NAFLD and the cellular mechanisms underlying hepatic lipids toxicity and its role in liver injury were elaborated. The contribution of HDL-C as a molecular modulator and the therapeutic implications of this knowledge were also discussed.

2. Molecular mechanisms and pathogenesis of NAFLD

It is essential to understand the processes that lead to NAFLD and NASH development. Even with the current advancement, our understanding of the pathogenesis of NAFLD is still lacking. The initial theory for the pathophysiology of NAFLD was based on two hypotheses. The first hypothesis described the accumulation of hepatic triglycerides which makes the liver more vulnerable to injury, mediated by the second hypothesis, such as inflammatory cytokines and adipokines, mitochondrial dysfunction, and oxidative stress, which in turn cause steatohepatitis and fibrosis. Also, an increased influx of free fatty acids (FFA) to the liver has been observed in IR and obesity. This concept, however, has been altered as FFA is increasingly understood to play a direct role in triggering liver injury [4, 6, 7]. The FFA can also promote hepatic lipid accumulation either through β-oxidation or esterified with glycerol to form triglycerides. Since convincing evidence has suggested that FFA can trigger inflammatory pathways by facilitating oxidative stress, hepatic triglyceride formation may serve as a defensive

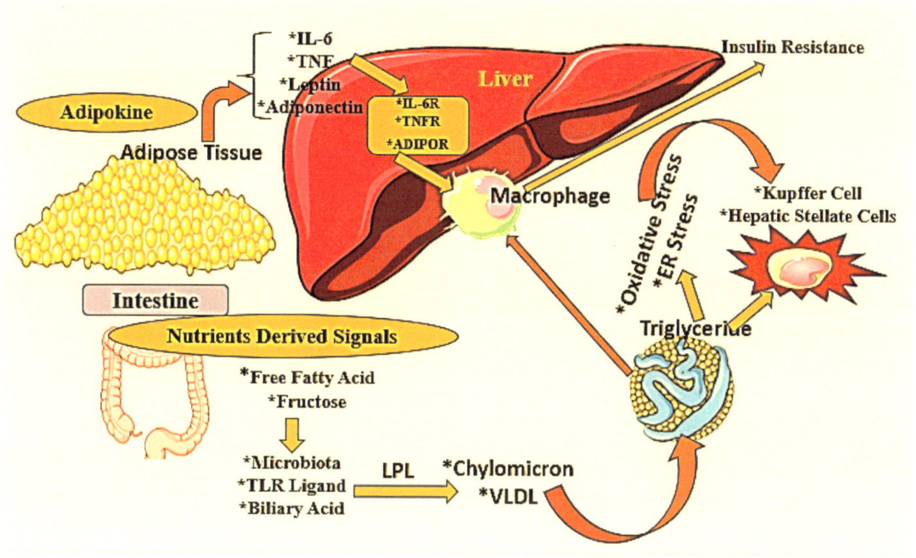

Figure 1.
Molecular mechanisms of NAFLD progression. Lipid accumulation and and high cholesterol levels can lead to alterations in intestinal flora, insulin resistance, and adipocyte proliferation. Free fatty acid and free cholesterol consumption leads to ER stress, oxidative stress, hepatic inflammation, and fibrogenesis, which promotes the development of NAFLD. Adipocytes secrete adipokines including IL-6 and TNF, which have an impact on the liver inflammatory environment and hepatocyte fat accumulation. Macrophages are crucial in the development of inflammation and insulin resistance. Recent study has recognized the gut microbiome as being associated with the development of NAFLD. The pattern of microbiome diversity can facilitate intestinal mucosal permeability and lead to lipopolysaccharidaemia, which is correlated with the development of NAFLD and NASH. Lipoprotein lipase (LPL) activity and triglyceride accumulation are both increased when enteric bacteria inhibit the secretion of adipocyte factor.

mechanism to counteract the harmful effects of unesterified FFA. In a healthy liver, apoptotic cells prompt mature hepatocytes to multiply, replacing the dead cells and re-establishing normal tissue function [4]. However, oxidative stress, a key factor in the development of NAFLD, prevents mature hepatocytes from replicating, which causes the population of hepatic progenitor cells to increase. The hepatic progenitor cells can differentiate into hepatocyte-like cells, and together with intermediate hepatocyte-like cells, can have numbers that are strongly correlated with the fibrosis stage, signifying that cumulative hepatocyte loss stimulates both the deposition of progenitor cells and their differentiation into hepatocytes. Hepatocellular carcinogenesis has also been linked to the activation of these cells. Since the effectiveness of hepatocyte regeneration is required for the fibrosis and cirrhosis that results from chronic liver injury, cell death with impaired hepatocyte progenitor proliferation is thought to be the "third hypothesis" in the pathogenesis of NAFLD [4]. Several factors, including oxidative stress, insulin resistance, steatohepatitis, endoplasmic reticulum stress, bacterial overgrowth, fibrosis, genetic implications, immune system, and beverages consumption, have been implicated in the progress of NAFLD (**Figure 1**) [4].

2.1 Contribution of oxidative stress and mitochondrial dysfunction in NAFLD formation

The influences of oxidative stress and mitochondrial dysfunction in NAFLD and NASH are well-recognized. Within the normal liver, β-oxidation occurs in the mitochondria but in the setting of NAFLD, this process can become overwhelmed due to elevated FFA load, leading to the generation of ROS. ROS stimulate oxidative stress with a progressive activation of mitochondrial damage and inflammatory pathways [8, 9]. Oxidative stress defines the imbalance between the production of ROS and the scavenging capacity of the antioxidant system to counteract the effect of the ROS produced. A high concentration of ROS intensifies the modifications of cellular macromolecules, such as DNA, proteins and lipids, which could lead to the deposition of damaged macromolecules and subsequently induce liver injury. Hence, the mechanism by which ROS contribute to NAFLD development may be associated with deregulated redox signaling and undifferentiating oxidative biomolecular injury (**Figure 2**) [9]. While the hepatic detoxification process in the liver serves as the main cause of oxidative stress, the biotransformation responses and physiologically generate intermediate ROS to permit the oxidation of toxins and promote their detoxification and excretion. Thus, under normal situations, the levels of ROS generated are the actual amounts needed for the normal body detoxification process and the body system syntheses many antioxidant cofactors that are essentially needed to counterbalance the generation of ROS [4, 6, 7]. On the other hand, insufficient production of endogenous antioxidant molecules and overloading of toxins may facilitate oxidative stress, which in turn may enhance tissue injury and promote the

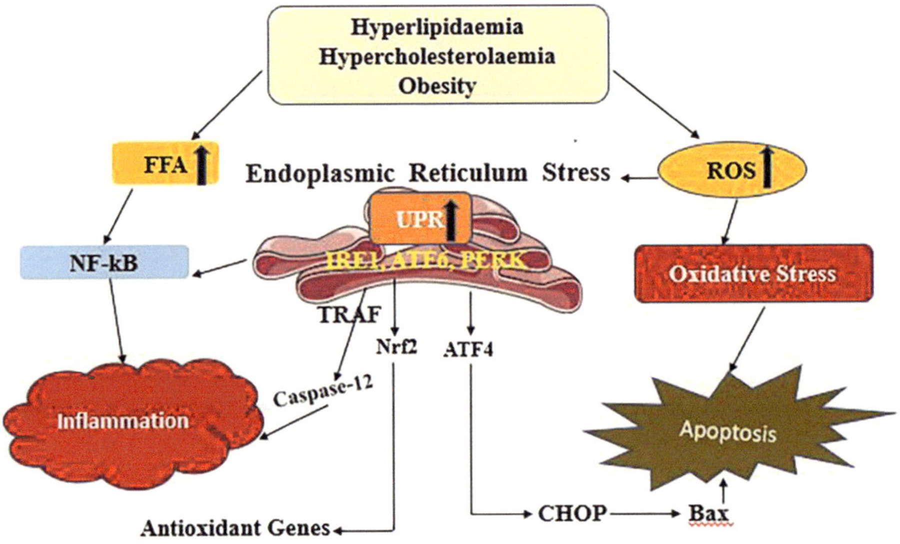

Figure 2.
Mechanisms of endoplasmic reticulum stress induced-NAFLD. NAFLD is associated with deposition of lipids in the liver, on which lipids promote several cellular stress pathways, such as ER stress and oxidative stress. ER stress enhances UPR which is facilitated by the activation of ER proteins, including ATF6, IRE1 and PERK. Through the phosphorylation of Nrf2, which controls the transcription of antioxidant genes, PERK activation enhances the defense against oxidative stress. Additionally, PERK promotes ATF4, which in turn triggers the transcription of CHOP and controls apoptosis through the Bax protein. Apoptosis results through an interaction between activated IRE1 and TRAF2 and complex recruits Caspase-12. When ER stress is maintained by increasing FFA, PERK and ATF-6 sensors can also activate NF-kB. Additionally, hyperlipidaemia, hypercholesterolemia and obesity can raise the amount of ROS that trigger apoptosis through oxidative stress pathways. Oxidative stress and ER stress are correlated in a bidirectional manner. ATF: Activating transcription factor, CHOP: C/EBP-homologous protein, FFA: Free fatty acid, IRE1: Inositol requiring enzyme-1, NF-κB: Nuclear factor κ-light-chain-enhancer of activated B cells, Nrf2: Nuclear factor 2 erythroid 2-related factor, PERK: Protein kinase RNA-like ER kinase, ROS; reactive oxygen species, TRAF2: TNF-α receptor-associated factor 2.

inflammation process [2, 5]. Furthermore, oxidative stress has progressively shown to be one of the major essential pathological processes in the development of NAFLD and the relationship between NASH manifestation and simple steatosis. Oxidative stress has been attributed to various chronic disorders, particularly those associated with low-grade inflammation, including DM, obesity and other metabolic syndromes [2, 5]. Oxidative stress has also been investigated as the major factor associated with the pathophysiology and development of CVDs and was suggested to be a possible mechanism, that links NAFLD to CVDs. While CVDs represent the leading cause of global death and morbidity, in this respect, only a few NAFLD patients may have chronic liver disease. Another important cellular source of oxidative stress is NADPH oxidase (Nox) and its stimulation has been linked with the possible progress of liver injury. The NADPH oxidase family, such as Nox1, Nox2, and Nox4, were suggested to control the activation of hepatic apoptosis and HSCs, which are essential in the fibrogenic process [2, 4, 5].

2.2 Endoplasmic reticulum stress

Endoplasmic reticulum (ER) stress is another pathway associated with the pathophysiology of NAFLD and NASH [10]. Unfolded proteins can accumulate within the ER, due to the increased protein synthesis input, the dysfunctional ER or a lack of ATP, which can activate the so-called "unfolded protein response (UPR)," an adaptive response designed to alleviate ER stress [11]. To identify the protein-folding defect that would otherwise result in the onset of apoptosis, UPR activation involves adaptive mechanisms such as reduction of protein synthesis, increased capacity for protein transit through the ER (**Figure 2**), increased protein folding and transport, and activation of pathways for protein degradation. The ER stress has been explained by various biological stresses, including hyperlipidaemia, hyperinsulinemia, high blood sugar, hypercholesterolaemia, oxidative stress, mitochondrial damage that depletes ATP, and low phosphatidylcholine levels. These can facilitate various pathways that could lead to mitochondrial dysfunction, IR, inflammation and apoptosis, which have been considered as the major factors that cause UPR in NAFLD [6, 8]. UPR has been identified to stimulate c-junk terminal kinase (JNK), a potent enhancer of inflammation and apoptosis. Although the activity of JNK was suggested to differentiate between patients with NASH from those with simple steatosis, its silencing in animal models suppresses both steatosis and steatohepatitis. JNK activity is also linked with decreased insulin signaling, which could initiate the episode of DM. Future research on the consequence of ER stress in NAFLD and NASH is important because it was investigated to have a significant implication on alcohol-induced steatohepatitis [6].

2.3 Insulin resistance

In healthy individuals, insulin receptor substrates (IRS), among other substrates, are phosphorylated when it binds to its receptor, which transmits the insulin signal [4]. Insulin resistance is among the major causes of NAFLD, which increases hepatic lipogenesis and inhibits adipose tissue lipolysis, resulting in an enhanced influx of fatty acids into the liver. Hepatocytes store fat mostly in the form of triglycerides generated by the esterification of glycerol and FFAs. Hepatic accumulation of triglyceride functions as a defense mechanism to balance off the excess FFAs in the plasma rather than as a hepatotoxic event. However, diacylglycerol (DAG) and other bioactive intermediates, such as ceramides, can cause lipotoxicity, which may progress to inflammation, necrosis, and hepatic fibrosis [12]. When the mechanisms protecting hepatocytes against lipotoxicity are depleted, NAFLD develops into NASH. This causes necrosis, secondary repair processes, and accumulation of scar collagen tissue, which are controlled by hepatic stellate cells, leading to the progress and development of hepatic fibrosis. Insulin resistance is also associated with hyperinsulinemia, which can result in the upregulation of transcription factor sterol regulatory element binding protein-1c (SREBP-1c), a major transcriptional regulator of genes involved in DNL and the inhibition of FFA's β-oxidation, which could further promote the deposition of hepatic lipids. Several anomalies investigated in NAFLD inhibit the insulin signaling pathway, which in turn causes IR. Elevated lipid metabolites, including diacylglycerol (DAG), have been linked to a protein kinase C (PKC) dependent process that blocks insulin receptor activation and insulin signaling modifies IRS-2 phosphorylation [13].

2.4 Inflammation and steatohepatitis

Hepatic steatosis in NAFLD is primarily caused by systemic insulin resistance, while NASH is majorly caused by lipotoxicity of accumulating lipids and innate immune system activation. Inflammatory mechanisms, such as the production of proinflammatory extracellular vesicles and cell death, are activated due to lipid-induced sub-lethal and lethal stress [1, 14]. Steatosis and chronic hepatic inflammation are strongly linked to NAFLD, and the Iκκ-β/NF-κB signaling pathway is partially responsible for this association. FFA can directly activate the Ikk-/BNF-kB pathway in hepatocytes, providing another mechanism through which central obesity and the resultant increase in hepatic FFA supply promote inflammation (**Figures 1** and **2**). Additionally, the transformation of FFA into hepatic triglyceride might act to protect against the direct toxicity of lipoproteins to the liver. Existing evidence has demonstrated that the suppression of DGAT2, the enzyme that catalyzes the last stage in triglyceride synthesis, improved hepatic steatosis and IR while exacerbating damage and fibrosis in a mouse model of NAFLD [15].

2.5 Fibrosis

Hepatocellular carcinoma, fibrosis and its more severe form, hepatic cirrhosis represent a final common pathway of most chronic liver diseases, such as NAFLD and NASH. Fibrosis is caused by excessive secretion of extracellular matrix (ECM) that is not sufficiently balanced by degradation, leading to a net accumulation. In the models of toxic, biliary liver disease and NAFLD, hepatic stellate cells (HSC) are the primary source of ECM-producing fibroblasts [16]. Twenty genetically distinct types of fibrillary and non-fibrillar collagen, as well as non-collagenous glycoproteins-like elastin, laminin, and fibronectin, as well as glycosaminoglycans-like hyaluronan and proteoglycans, including aggrecan, fibromodulin, decorin, biglycan, glypicans, and syndecans, are all contained in the complex network of the ECM proteins. Together with increased amounts, the composition of the ECM proteins is also modified in fibrosis, leading to an increase in embryonic or wound-healing associated ECM and an increase in crosslinks that make the ECM more resistant to degradation, contributing to delay and incomplete reversibility of severe fibrosis. A more progressive pattern of liver damage may be caused by an inability to develop a ductular response, as seen in patients with denervated liver, who have undergone liver transplantation for NASH [16].

2.6 Bacterial overgrowth

Existing evidence points to the involvement of bacterial overgrowth in the pathogenesis of NAFLD and NASH. The gut microbiome is implicated in the pathogenesis and progression of NAFLD through the so-called gut-liver axis, investigating that the gut microbiome could be considered a metabolic organ in the host, which can affect human metabolism in health and disease [13]. Bacterial overgrowth results in the secretion of bacterial lipopolysaccharides (LPS), which can activate the production of TNF-α, and ethanol. Bacterial LPS are produced when Gram-negative bacteria proliferate excessively and are mostly transported due to increased intestinal permeability. Furthermore, the interaction between LPS and the Toll-like receptors (TLRs4) system increases oxidative stress in NAFLD because of the excessive ROS generation and deficiency in endogenous antioxidant molecules [7]. Oxidative stress has also been reported to be overexpressed in CVDs, which may be a link that connects LPS to the elevated cardiovascular risk in NAFLD patients. The elevated LPS levels in the circulation may result from various factors. In the intestine, the absorption of LPS together with chylomicrons intensifies the chance of NAFLD development, which is activated by hepatic inflammatory cells. Additionally, intestinal bacteria stimulate lipoprotein lipase activity and triglyceride accumulation by inhibiting the synthesis of fasting-induced adipocyte factor (FIAF) [7]. Furthermore, the gut microbiota syntheses enzymes that facilitate the transformation of dietary choline into toxic substances, such as methylamines, which can be utilized by the liver, transformed into trimethylamine-N-oxide, and subsequently promote inflammation and liver damage. Also, bacterial endotoxins have damaging effects on hepatocytes and can stimulate Kupffer cells to generate inflammatory cytokines, which would then cause the waterfall effect and the generation of oxygen radicals [6, 7]. TLRs on hepatocytes, HSCs, and Kupfer cells detect bacterial endotoxins. Signaling of bacterial LPS through TLR4 activates the nuclear factor kappa-light-chain-enhancer of activated B cells (NF-kB) (**Figures 1** and 2) and subsequent inflammasome activation. Increased secretion of bile acids (Bas) facilitated by a high-fat diet is another mechanism that may result in gut hyperpermeability in individuals with NAFLD. Gut permeability is compromised because of BAs, which increase epidermal growth receptor (EGFR) activity. Generally, these pathways could partially account for the "leaky gut" phenomenon seen in the majority of NAFLD patients [6, 7, 13].

2.7 Glucocorticoids (GCs)

GCs sources from both exogenous and endogenous have been recognized to be implicated in NAFLD development. Individuals with Cushing's syndrome, who have elevated GCs levels are associated with characteristic metabolic phenotype, including IR, central obesity, and DM, and many of these patients will have hepatic steatosis. Inhibition of fatty acid β-oxidation and activation of hepatocyte DNL have been reported as the potential mechanisms through which GCs stimulate hepatic lipid accumulation. Still, several individuals will have normal cortisol levels, indicating that tissue-specific pathways are involved in this metabolic dysfunction [4].

2.8 Involvement of the immune system

Innate immune cells play a crucial role in the pathogenesis of NAFLD [5]. Although the innate immune system is activated and proinflammatory monocytes are recruited into the liver in NASH, the precise signals that result from this are still poorly understood [17, 18]. Increased FFA levels, which result in lipotoxicity, insulin resistance, dysfunctional peripheral adipose tissue, and endotoxins originating from the gut, contribute to activating and maintaining the synthesis and release of pro-inflammatory cytokines in the liver at both local and systemic levels. JNK-AP-1 and IKK-NF-kB are two major inflammatory pathways that play a crucial role in the emergence of the chronic inflammatory state in NAFLD [6]. *In vitro* experiments employing cultured HepG2 cells and primary mouse, hepatocytes show that the release of damage-associated molecular patterns (DAMPs) from hepatocytes activates innate immune cells, especially macrophages (Kupffer cells). Additionally, several specific DAMPs, including high-mobility-group protein box 1 (HMGB1), have been demonstrated to activate TLR4 in NASH and NAFLD, playing a crucial role in the initial setting of NAFLD. In humans, other DAMPs, such as sonic hedgehog (SHH) ligands, have also been linked to the development of NAFLD and fibrosis. Another important component of NAFLD and NASH is neutrophils. The protease neutrophil elastase (NE), which is synthesized by neutrophils, secretes cellular IR, while deletion of NE results in less tissue inflammation [5]. Increased concentration of blood from the gut to the portal vein exposed the liver to gut-derived endotoxin, leading to endotoxemia, which activates Kupffer cells through the TLR4 complex on the cell surface. The Toll-like family of pattern recognition receptors are crucial for host defense against invading pathogens. When endotoxin interacts with TLR-4, a variety of proinflammatory mediators are released, leading to hepatic fibrosis and damage. Furthermore, cytokines have a significant impact on lipid metabolism [19]. Chitotriosidase (CHIT), an enzyme from the glycosylhydrolase family, is one of the mechanisms associated with the immune response in NASH and NAFLD. The CHIT gene spans around 20 kb of genomic DNA and is found on chromosome 1q31–q32 and has 12 exons. The majority of freshly generated 50 kDa CHIT is secreted by tissue macrophages, and a subsequent step cleaves the enzyme to secrete the active form of CHIT (39 kDa). Pathological tissue macrophages massively express CHIT in many conditions. In humans, NASH patients have much greater levels of CHIT expression than NAFLD patients or control subjects, which indicates a direct relationship between CHIT expression and the severity of NASH. Hence, patients with NASH had greater plasma levels of CHIT activity than those with NAFLD [20].

2.9 Genetic implication

Identification of genetic factors to determine the risk of disease progression may assist to evaluate individuals who may have associated morbidity. Various genes associated with NAFLD have been investigated but the most frequent variant; p.I148M of the enzyme adiponectin gene is one of the major genetic determinants of steatosis and steatohepatitis, fibrosis, cirrhosis, and hepatocellular cancer [2]. Furthermore, polymorphism in the TM6SF2 gene (rs58542926c.449 C > T, p.Glu167Lys) has been associated with severe hepatic fibrosis and cirrhosis, but the underlying mechanisms responsible for these gene variants to influence liver damage are still lacking [2]. In addition to environmental factors, genes also affect NAFLD and through the genome-wide association analyses, several genes have been discovered, on which transmembrane 6 superfamily member 2 (TM6SF2) and patatin-like phospholipase domain containing 3 (PNPLA3) appear to be more implicated. Triacylglycerol hydrolysis is mediated by a 481 amino acid protein that is encoded by the PNPLA3 gene, which is found on chromosome 22. PNPLA3's

I148M variant (rs738409), is substantially linked to NAFLD in adults, as well as obese kids and teenagers, although the precise mechanism is still unknown. The TM6SF2 gene, which is found on chromosome 19, contributes to the development of NAFLD. A single nucleotide polymorphism (rs58542926) that replaces the position 167 of cytosine to thymine has been associated with an elevated hepatic triglyceride level. The development of fibrosis has also been linked to this gene variant and the effects of PNLPA3 and TM6SF2 on NASH and severe fibrosis are cumulative [21]. Only a small percentage of people with obesity and IR develop NASH and cirrhosis, even though hepatic steatosis is widespread in these patients, indicating an essential interaction between genetic predisposition and environmental factors. NAFLD and NASH formations may be made more susceptible by polymorphisms in genes involved in lipid metabolism, IR, oxidative stress, cytokines, and fibrogenesis. Single nucleotide polymorphisms (SNPs) that affect fibrosis development in various liver diseases, including chronic hepatitis C, have been found in several reports. Existing evidence has shown that angiotensinogen and TGF-1 gene polymorphisms have been linked to progressive liver fibrosis in obese patients with NAFLD and NASH. Also, NAFLD and NAFLD-related fibrosis are linked to SNPs in the angiotensin II type 1 receptor [4].

2.10 Influences of beverages in non-alcoholic fatty liver disease

The most popular types of alcoholic drinks include wines, beers, and spirits, whereas non-alcoholic drinks include juices, carbonated and non-carbonated sweetened drinks, and hot beverages like tea and coffee. Even though certain drinks provide fundamental health advantages, beverages are regarded as functional foods because they include well-known macro- or micro-molecules that support optimal health. Independent of the metabolic syndrome, soft drink use can raise the prevalence of NAFLD. Regular soft drink consumption causes the primary effect of fructose, which increases lipogenesis. The additional contribution of aspartame sweetener and caramel colorant, which are rich in advanced glycation end products, may increase insulin resistance and inflammation. Hence, lipids accumulation in the liver can result from regular soft drink consumption [22, 23]. Consuming sugar-sweetened drinks (SSBs) is also linked to increased triglyceride levels, abdominal fat, blood pressure, IR and lower HDL cholesterol levels, which may facilitate the development of NAFLD and obesity. Despite the negative effects of sugar-sweetened beverages and energy drinks, there is some evidence that drinking tea, coffee, and alcoholic beverages may have some positive effects on liver disease. SSBs increase hepatic de novo lipogenesis while reducing fatty acid β-oxidation, which in turn promotes NAFLD. Despite the lifestyle factors, obesity, CVDs and metabolic syndrome, increased deposition of visceral and hepatic fat are the main risk factors linked to daily consumption of sugar-sweetened beverages [24, 25]. Several mechanisms have been investigated to show how fructose might participate in the production of lipids in the liver. Fructose has also been investigated to facilitate hepatic lipid deposition through the dysfunctional mitochondria and mitigate β-oxidation of fatty acids. Another significant component of SSB is glucose, which can either directly or indirectly stimulate hepatic lipid storage by converting into fructose through the polyol pathway in the liver [22]. Moreover, fructose may activate the lipogenic transcription factors sterol receptor element binding protein 1c (SREBP-1c) and carbohydrate response element binding protein (ChREBP). Fructose may limit the breakdown of fatty acids by lowering the activity of β-oxidation in the liver as another mechanism. Numerous studies have demonstrated that SSB consumption may raise the risk of hyperuricemia by depleting adenosine triphosphate (ATP), which may then increase alanine aminotransferase (ALT) levels [25].

3. Modulation of liver injury in NAFLD by HDL

The hepato-protective activity of HDL in the body is tightly related to its function in facilitating cholesterol efflux, determined by CEC through various pathways [26].

3.1 Lipid metabolism and significant of HDL

Lipid metabolism involves several key enzymes and subtypes of lipid fractions and lipoproteins. These include lipoprotein lipase (LPL), TGs, TC, LDL, VLDL, HDL, and chylomicrons (**Figure 3**). Lipid metabolism formed the cornerstone for understanding the mechanisms involved in the atherothrombotic formation. Lipid metabolism occurs through three essential pathways, including exogenous and endogenously produced lipids, and finally the reverse cholesterol transport pathway (**Figure 3**) [27, 28]. The exogenous (dietary) pathway begins with chylomicron synthesis and secretion by the intestine. Dietary fat and cholesterol are absorbed by the duodenum and proximal jejunum. In the intestinal duodenum, dietary lipids undergo emulsification and then

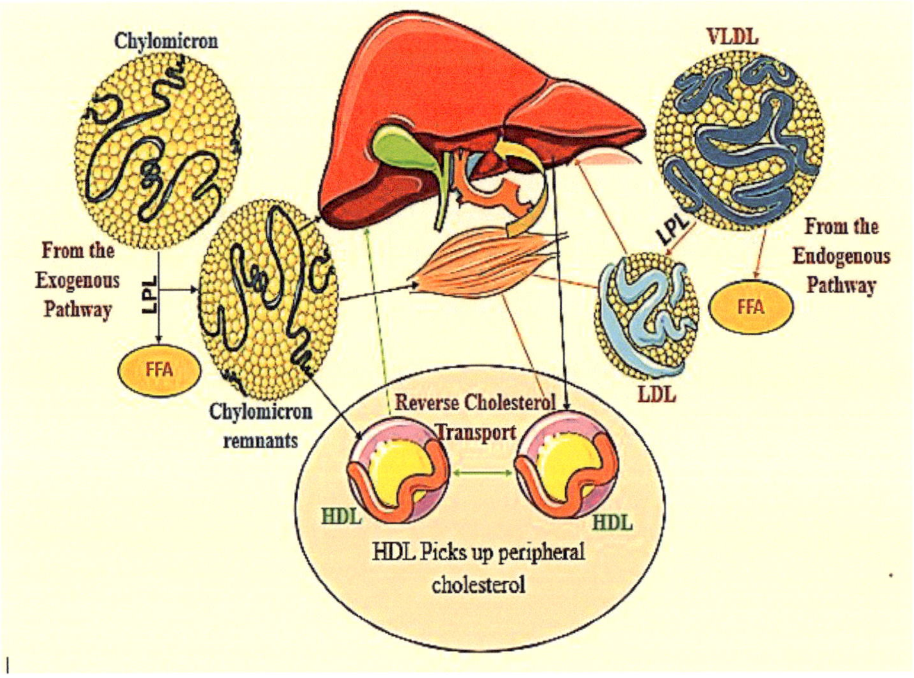

Figure 3.
Mechanism of reverse cholesterol transport (RCT): From the exogenous pathway, LPL acts on chylomicrons to generate FFAs, while the chylomicron remnant are transported to the liver. In the endogenous pathway, the LPL cleaves VLDL to form IDLs, which are utilized by the liver. The reverse cholesterol transport pathway involves the action of HDL, which picks up the peripheral cholesterols and returns them to the liver for recycling. LPL; lipoprotein lipase, FFAs; free fatty acids, HDL; high-density lipoproteins, VLDL; very low-density lipoprotein, LDL; low-density lipoprotein, IDL; intermediate lipoprotein.

hydrolysed by the pancreatic and intestinal lipases. Hydrolysis products, such as free fatty acids and monoglycerides are then transferred to the intestinal epithelial cell, where they diffuse through the epithelial cell membranes into the intestinal mucosal cells. In the small intestinal mucosal cells, free fatty acids and monoglycerides reassemble to form triglycerides, which then combine with proteins, phospholipids, free and esterified cholesterol to form Chylomicrons [29]. Chylomicrons are the lipoprotein class responsible for dietary lipids transport. After their formation in the enterocytes, chylomicrons, which mainly contain triglycerides, are secreted into the lacteals and enter into the blood circulation through the lymphatic system. Chylomicrons contain apolipoproteins (Apos) B-48, C-II, and E. The Apo C-II is an essential co-factor of lipoprotein lipase (LPL) during the transportation of fatty acids to adipose tissue. After LPL activity, the chylomicron remnant is relatively enriched in cholesterol due to the loss of triacylglycerol and absorbed into the liver by Apo E [30]. Lipoprotein, which is exposed on the chylomicron surface, activates the lipoprotein lipase attached to the capillary beds in adipose and skeletal muscle tissues, which then hydrolyses triglycerides into free fatty acids (FFAs) and glycerol. The FFAs enter the muscle cells, where they are used for energy production and to the adipocytes, where they would be re-esterified into triglycerides for storage. The chylomicron remnants return to HDL to be recycled by the liver and are recognized by specific hepatic receptors that rapidly remove them from the circulation by endocytosis. The cholesterol found in chylomicron remnants can be used for VLDL, bile acid formation, or stored as cholesteryl esters [28]. While the chylomicrons are responsible for the transport of dietary lipids, endogenously synthesized triglycerides, cholesterols and cholesteryl esters, including VLDL, LDL and HDL are mainly involved in the endogenous lipid metabolism pathway. The endogenous pathway starts with the synthesis of VLDL particles, which are triglyceride-rich and contain Apo B-100, C-II, and E. After the removal of the triglycerides in adipose tissue, a portion of VLDL remnants is metabolized to LDL particles [30]. Thus, VLDL remnants are either removed from the circulation by the liver or undergo further transformation by lipoprotein lipase or hepatic lipase to form LDL. As LPL cleaves TGs, the cholesterol concentration within the lipoprotein increases and becomes a smaller denser lipoprotein named "intermediate-density lipoproteins" (IDL) [27]. The IDL can be taken up by the liver through an apoE-dependent process, while LDL is taken up by the liver through the binding of apoB100 to LDL receptors. The LDL which mainly contains cholesteryl esters and phospholipids circulates in the blood and binds to specific receptors that are widely distributed throughout the tissues. The small VLDL, IDL, and LDL particles may be taken up by peripheral tissues to deliver nutrients, cholesterol, and fat-soluble vitamins, to be used for the synthesis of steroid hormones and cell membranes as well as for hepatic metabolism [31].

HDL is a mixture of lipoproteins associated with various minor lipids and proteins that stimulates the function of HDL. Most of the HDL particles arise from lipid-free or poorly lipidated apoA-I secreted by hepatocytes and the intestinal mucosa or dissociated from lipolyzed chylomicrons and VLDL as well as from interconverting mature HDL particles [32]. The interaction between the lipid-free or poorly lipidated apoA-I, also known as the pre-β1-HDL with the ATP-binding cassette transporter A1 (ABCA1) leads to efflux of phospholipids and unesterified cholesterol from various cells, such as hepatocytes, enterocytes, and macrophages, which progress to the formation of small discoidal HDL particles, known as α_4-HDL. The α_4-HDL precursors can further facilitate the lipid efflux from cells, basically from scavenger receptor BI (SR-BI) or ATP-binding cassette transporter G1 (ABCG1) [2]. The effluxed cholesterol and phosphatidylcholine function as substrates of lecithin-cholesterol acyltransferase (LCAT) to generate water-insoluble cholesteryl esters, which transform to the core mature spherical HDL. The initial small α-HDL3 particles develop into larger α-HDL2 particles obtained from phospholipids and cholesterol from both cells (SR-BI or ABCG1), which is involved with the activity of phospholipid transfer protein, and apoB-containing lipoproteins fused with other HDL particles. The breaking down of HDL varies from that of LDL since only a minor proportion of HDL would be removed by holo-particle uptake into cells. In this poorly understood pathway, a high-affinity interaction of apoA-I with ectopic F0F1–ATPase leads to the generation of ADP, which stimulates purinergic receptors to facilitate the uptake of HDL by an as-yet-unidentified low-affinity HDL receptor [2, 32]. These pathways (**Figure 3**) promote the elimination of lipids from HDL irrespective of their protein content. The cholesteryl ester transfer protein (CETP) converts triglycerides of apoB-containing lipoproteins for cholesteryl esters of HDL, which are finally removed through the LDL receptor pathway, while SR-BI coordinates the uptake of HDL lipids into the liver and steroidogenic organs [8]. The elimination of cholesteryl esters by CETP and SR-BI, and the lipolysis of triglycerides and phospholipids by hepatic lipase and endothelial lipase, respectively, promote the transformation of HDL2 to HDL3, and the ultimate formation of pre-β1-HDL. This lipid-poor apoA-I either transforms to a mature HDL by activating ABCA1-mediated lipid efflux from several cells or is filtrated by the renal glomeruli through the proximal tubule of the kidneys. The apoA-I is endocytosed by the cubilin and megalin receptors and targeted for lysosomal degradation [32].

3.2 Reverse cholesterol transport (RCT)

Existing studies have investigated that extracellular levels, HDL molecular content and the activities of ABC transporter determine the cholesterol efflux. Also, previous reports have indicated that cellular cholesterol homeostasis, HDL-mediated efflux together with ABCG1 and cholesterol efflux by apoA-I/ ABCA1 plays a significant regulatory step in several cellular activities, such as proliferation, differentiation and mobilization of haemopoietic cells [26]. The RCT described a mechanism by which the body removes excess cholesterol from peripheral cells and tissues and delivers it to the liver after conversion to bile acids. The cholesterol will then be redistributed to other tissues or excreted from the body through the gallbladder, or to adrenals, testes, and ovaries for the synthesis of steroid hormones. Because cholesterol could not be metabolized by peripheral tissues, it must be transported back to the liver for removal through a pathway known as "reverse cholesterol transport" (**Figure 3**) determined by the HDL and its precursors [29]. The HDL-C is the main lipoprotein involved in this process, followed by the intestine, while the liver produces the protein Apo A-1 (70% of the protein content of HDL-c), which passes through the bloodstream and goes to peripheral tissues, such as the heart. In the circulation, Apo A-1 interacts with receptors in several cell types, including hepatocytes, enterocytes, and macrophages, known as ATP-Binding Cassette, Sub-Family A, Member 1 (ABCA1) [33]. In macrophages, the immune system specialized in phagocytosing particles, the interaction with this protein forces the cholesterols and some phospholipids to move toward the molecule Apo A-1. This interaction leads to the formation of nascent HDL-c particles (pre-b HDL), which can subsequently interact with scavenger receptor class B member 1 (SR-B1) and ATP-binding cassette, sub-family G, member 1 (ABCG1), and then incorporate more cholesterol to form a mature molecule of HDL-C (α-HDL), catalyzed by the enzyme LCAT. Cholesterols are delivered to the liver in both direct and indirect ways. In a direct way, mature molecules of HDL-C interact with SR-B1 in the liver, which permits the transfer of its cholesterol content, and the resulting HDL-C molecule can enter circulation and initiate another RCT process. The mature molecules of HDL-C can indirectly transfer its cholesterol content to apolipoproteins B-100 (Apo B-100), particularly to the LDL, in exchange for triacylglycerol molecules, a process catalyzed by the enzyme CETP, and hence, these lipoproteins can be linked with their liver receptors and deliver their cholesterol content. The CETP was also identified to catalyze the reverse transference, i.e., triacylglycerol from HDL-C in exchange for Apo B-100 cholesterol. The reduction in the synthesis of hepatic cholesterol leads to increased hepatic LDL-receptors, which bind and reduces the synthesis of circulating LDL and its precursors; IDL and VLDL [34]. The HDL cholesterol content in plasma may therefore be a crucial modulator to treat and prevent NAFLD since this molecule exerts anti-inflammatory functions as well as positive effects on CRT. Furthermore, recent studies have suggested that the functionality of HDL-c shows a much greater potential in some conditions, including dyslipidaemia and NAFLD [32, 35].

4. Current therapeutic target

The information above pointed out the various pathways associated with NAFLD pathogenesis and the role of HDL as a molecular modifier of NAFLD. Finding the most effective therapeutic targets is now much easier, due to our growing understanding of the pathophysiology of NAFLD. Indeed, correction and management of established NAFLD and NASH-associated factors implicated with the pathogenesis and progression, including excessive dietary energy and fructose intake, the extent of obesity, hyperlipidaemia, degree of IR, DM and oxidative stress are the current therapeutic targets of NAFLD and NASH treatment [2]. The current therapies available are projected toward improving the factors that suppress the disease pathogenesis, including exercise, weight loss, modification of lifestyle, decreasing IR and promoting DM control. At end-stage cirrhosis, liver transplant appears to be the only treatment option. Therapies that can cure or prevent fibrosis are essential in this regard because it is known that the existence of fibrosis in NAFLD is linked with other liver-associated complications [4]. Antioxidants, such as vitamins C, E, and betaine, iron depletion, statins, and pentoxifylline are some of the current treatments being evaluated in NAFLD and NASH. Others, including Glucagon-like peptide-1 (GLP-1)-based therapy, may be an advanced therapeutic alternative to inhibit the development of NAFLD. Drugs like exenatide, have been demonstrated to boost insulin secretion, inhibit glucagon secretion, suppress gastric emptying, and promote satiety with weight loss, demonstrated in both animal models and DM individuals [2]. Since angiotensin has been demonstrated to encourage myofibroblast survival and liver fibrosis, angiotensin-converting enzyme (ACE) inhibitors and angiotensin receptor blockers (ARBs) are anticipated to have significant effects, such as antifibrotic. The proliferative, contractile, and fibrogenic activities of HSCs are closely regulated by a wide number of cytokines, whose antagonistic effects constitute another possible target for antifibrotic treatments [27]. Platelet-derived growth factor (PDGF), transforming growth factor beta-1 (TGF-β1), connective tissue growth factor (CTGF), endothelin-1 (ET-1), thrombin, vascular endothelial growth factor (VEGF), fibroblast growth factor, and insulin-like growth factor are potential candidates, that exert their effects through tyrosine-kinase receptors [4]. Additionally, inhibiting ER stress and modifying the gut-liver axis utilizing pre- and probiotics are two other possible targets. A Mediterranean diet has been shown to minimize oxidative stress, and high daily doses of vitamin E have been shown to cause the resolution of NASH in 36% of treated individuals. Silymarin reduced transaminase levels in NAFLD patients, and long-term use of the drug may help lessen fibrosis and halt the progression of liver disease in NAFLD and NASH patients [4].

4.1 Common HDL-C-raising drugs

Even though HDL is considered a promising biomarker and potential therapeutic target based on its epidemiological data and the effects of healthy HDL *in vitro* in endothelial cells and macrophages, as well as based on infusion studies of reconstituted HDL in patients with hypercholesterolemia [32], it would be assumed that HDL-C–raising drugs will become part of preventive armamentarium in the future. Therefore, it will be important to demonstrate that novel drugs not only increase HDL-C plasma levels but also improve HDL functions. Based on the inverse epidemiological association that linked HDL-C plasma levels with several adverse effects of CVDs, HDL-C has been recognized as a potential therapeutic target. As such, many drugs to increase HDL-C levels have been established and examined at basic and clinical levels [8, 32]. Various advanced agents and drugs associated with cholesterol metabolism have been established in clinical trials that may be used to treat NAFLD and NASH. The CETP inhibitors.is the most potent novel category of HDL-C-increasing drugs. CETP is a plasma protein that suppresses the movement of cholesterol esters from HDL to LDL, leading to a marked and consistent increase in the plasma HDL-C levels. The most common is the fibrates, which significantly decreased plasma triglyceride levels and elevate the HDL-C levels [8]. Niacin has been used to treat individuals with hyperlipidaemia by raising the HDL-C levels to about 15% and 30% while reducing the concentration of LDL-C and triglycerides ApoA-I contains 243 amino acids were identified to promote HDL anti-inflammatory activities in various animal models of atherosclerosis and NAFLD. Oral administration of apoA-I mimetic peptide of 4.3 and 7.14 mg/kg doses significantly enhances HDL functionality and the HDL inflammatory index [2, 8, 32].

4.2 Other evidence-based treatment alternatives

4.2.1 Coffee consumption and NAFLD

Coffee and other caffeinated beverages enhance intestinal barrier performance, promote hepatic autophagy, and prevent the activation of HSCs. Due to the antioxidant and antifibrotic properties of several physiologically active chemicals it possesses, coffee appears to be protective against many hepatic conditions, including liver fibrosis and cirrhosis. Coffee is also protective in people with NAFLD; due to the number of antioxidants as well as the caffeine itself, which has anti-inflammatory characteristics [6, 13]. The beneficial effect of decaffeinated coffee on the development of NASH was mediated through attenuating intestinal nitric oxide synthase (NOS) protein and restoration of intestinal barrier functioning, whereas the antifibrotic effect of coffee was exerted by caffeine-mediated antagonism of adenosine receptor which further leads to hepatic stellate cells inactivation. Chlorogenic acid, a key component of regular coffee, lowers the frequency of NAFLD perhaps by facilitating hepatic autophagy, enhancing gut barrier function, and reducing hepatic inflammation through the TLR4 pathway [22].

4.2.2 Tea consumption and NAFLD

Tea intake modulates NAFLD by suppressing inflammation and lipogenesis while promoting fatty acid β-oxidation. *Camellia sinensis* leaves and buds are used to make green and black tea, however, due to variations in post-harvest processing, their polyphenol content varies. Catechins (flavan-3-ols), which make up about 20% of the total flavonoids in green tea leaves are the main polyphenols and EGCG (Epigallocatechin gallate) [2, 22]. In humans, between the ages of 10 and 16, drinking green tea has been shown to lower plasma levels of aminotransferases, triglycerides, and improve BMI, explaining that drinking tea helps protect against NAFLD is supported by the tight association between these factors and NAFLD. *In-vivo* research has previously demonstrated that green tea has antioxidant capabilities, it reduces the accumulation of lipids in the liver and adipose tissue and prevents intestinal absorption of dietary lipids. In the mouse model of NAFLD, green tea extract (GTE) has been discovered to protect against hepatic steatosis and related liver damage. Recent research suggests that GTE therapy reduces pro-inflammatory signals through TLR4 and TNFR1, which in turn reduces inflammation in steatohepatitis [22]. Green tea catechins have also been demonstrated to support hepatic lipid metabolism. It was suggested that oxidative degradation of fatty acids by catechins acts as a protective mechanism against NAFLD and also functioning as a natural iron chelator. It has been found that giving patients EGCG reduces non-heme iron absorption by 27%. Since elevated hepatic iron levels have been linked to NASH in patients, while catechins that block iron absorption may be a useful treatment for NAFLD. Similar to this, theaflavin from black tea reduced liver steatosis, oxidative stress, inflammation, and apoptosis in mice with NAFLD-induced ischemia-reperfusion injury [22].

5. Conclusion

The mechanisms associated with the deposition and maintenance of excess hepatic lipids define an imbalance between the hepatic production and removal of TGs, which are majorly transferred from the liver within VLDLs. Data concerning which toxic lipids induce liver injury in NAFLD and NASH are limited. Agents or factors that stimulate or modulate liver damage in NAFLD can assist to identify potential therapeutic targets. HDLs have been recognized as good cholesterol, essential to the body, which functions to ameliorate various metabolic conditions, including CVDs and NAFLD. Correction and management of the factors involved in the pathophysiology and progression of NAFLD, including hyperlipidaemia, obesity, IR, DM, oxidative stress, lifestyle, inactivity and poor dietary control are the current therapeutic targets for NAFLD. To minimize liver damage in NAFLD, new approaches that target HDL-induced drugs and cholesterol metabolism pathways may be helpful in lowering hepatic cholesterol content.

Author details

Ibrahim Kalle Kwaifa[1*], Abdullahi S. Mainasara[2], Muhammad Lawal Jidda[3], Amrina Mohammad Amin[4], Garba Abdullahi[5], Faruku Ladan[6] and Maryam Danyaro[1]

1 Department of Haematology, Usmanu Danfodiyo University Teaching Hospital (UDUTH), Sokoto, North-Western, Nigeria

2 Department of Chemical Pathology, College of Health Sciences, Usmanu Danfodiyo University (UDU), Sokoto, North-Western, Nigeria

3 Department of Chemical Pathology, School of Medical Laboratory Sciences, College of Health Sciences, Usmanu Danfodiyo University (UDU), Sokoto, Nigeria

4 Faculty of Medicine and Health Sciences, Haematology Unit, Department of Pathology, Universiti Putra Malaysia (UPM), Seri Kembangan, Malaysia

5 Central Advanced Science Laboratory Complex, Usmanu Danfodiyo University (UDU), Sokoto, North-Western, Nigeria

6 Department of Chemical Pathology, Usmanu Danfodiyo University Teaching Hospital (UDUTH), Sokoto, North-Western, Nigeria

*Address all correspondence to: nanamarye2009@gmail.com

References

[1] Parthasarathy G, Revelo X, Malhi H. Pathogenesis of nonalcoholic steatohepatitis: An overview. Hepatology Communication. 2020;**4**(4):478-492. DOI: 10.1002/hep4.1479

[2] Arguello G, Balboa E, Arrese M, et al. Recent insights on the role of cholesterol in non-alcoholic fatty liver disease. Biochimica et Biophysica Acta (BBA)—Molecular Basis of Disease. 2015;**1852**:1765-1778

[3] Zou Y, Hu C, Kuang M, Chai Y. Remnant cholesterol/high-density lipoprotein cholesterol ratio is a new powerful tool for identifying non-alcoholic fatty liver disease. BMC Gastroenterology. 2022;**22**(1):134. DOI: 10.1186/s12876-022-02216-x

[4] Dowman JK, Tomlinson JW, Newsome PN. Pathogenesis of non-alcoholic fatty liver disease. QJM: An International Journal of Medicine. 2010;**103**(2):71-83. DOI: doi.org/10.1093/qjmed/hcp158

[5] Idalsoaga F, Kulkarni AV, Mousa OY, Arrese M, Arab JP. Non-alcoholic fatty liver disease and alcohol-related liver disease: Two intertwined entities. Frontiers in Medicine. 2020;**7**:448. DOI: 10.3389/fmed.2020.00448

[6] Buzzetti E, Pinzani M, Tsochatzis EA. The multiple-hit pathogenesis of non-alcoholic fatty liver disease (NAFLD). Metabolism. 2016;**65**(8):1038-1048. DOI: 10.1016/j.metabol.2015.12.012. Epub 2016 Jan 4

[7] Domenico F, Francesco B, Daniele P, Nicholas C, Alessandra C, Francesco A, et al. New insights into the pathogenesis of non-alcoholic fatty liver disease: Gut-derived lipopolysaccharides and oxidative stress. Nutrients. 2020;**12**:2762. DOI: 10.3390/nu12092762 6, 7

[8] Wang HH, Garruti G, Liu M, et al. Cholesterol and lipoprotein metabolism and atherosclerosis: Recent advances in reverse cholesterol transport. Annals of Hepatology. 2017;**16**:s27-s42

[9] Lüscher TF, Landmesser U, Von Eckardstein A, et al. High-density lipoprotein: Vascular protective effects, dysfunction, and potential as therapeutic target. Circulation Research. 2014;**114**:171-182

[10] Fadaei R, Poustchi H, Meshkani R, Moradi N, Golmohammadi T, Merat S. Impaired HDL cholesterol efflux capacity in patients with non-alcoholic fatty liver disease is associated with subclinical atherosclerosis. Scientific Reports. 3 Aug 2018;**8**(1):11691. DOI: 10.1038/s41598-018-29639-5

[11] World Health Organization (WHO). Raised Cholesterol-Global Health Obsevatory (GHO) data. 2020. Available from: https://www.who.int/gho/ncd/risk_fa

[12] Fan N, Peng L, Xia Z, et al. Triglycerides to high-density lipoprotein cholesterol ratio as a surrogate for nonalcoholic fatty liver disease: a cross-sectional study. Lipids Health Dis. 2019;**18**(1):39. Published 2019 Feb 2. DOI: 10.1186/s12944-019-0986-7

[13] Caturano A, Acierno C, Nevola R, Pafundi PC, Galiero R, Rinaldi L, et al. Non-Alcoholic fatty liver disease: From Pathogenesis to Clinical Impact. Processes. 2021;**9**(1):135. DOI: 10.3390/pr9010135

[14] Xiaoyan L, Hua W. Multiple organs involved in the pathogenesis of

non-alcoholic fatty liver disease. Cell & Bioscience. 2020;**10**:140

[15] Juan PA, Marco A, Michael T. Mechanisms of disease recent insights into the pathogenesis of nonalcoholic fatty liver disease. Annual Review of Pathology. 2018;**13**:321-350

[16] Schwabe RF, Ira T, Utpal BP. Mechanisms of fibrosis development in NASH. Gastroenterology. 2020;**158**(7):1913-1928. DOI: 10.1053/j.gastro.2019.11.311

[17] Pafili K, Roden M. Nonalcoholic fatty liver disease (NAFLD) from pathogenesis to treatment concepts in humans. Molecular Metabolism. Aug 2021; **50**:101122. DOI: 10.1016/j.molmet.2020.101122. Epub [19 Nov, 2020]

[18] Lang S, Schnabl B. Microbiota and fatty liver disease-the known, the unknown, and the future. Cell Host & Microbe. 2020;**28**(2):233-244. DOI: 10.1016/j.chom.2020.07.007

[19] Ilan Y. Leaky gut and the liver: A role for bacterial translocation in nonalcoholic steatohepatitis. World Journal of Gastroenterology. 2012;**18**(21):2609-2618. DOI: 10.3748/wjg. v18.i21.2609

[20] Norberto C, Chávez-Tapia M, Uribe G, Ponciano-Rodríguez R, Medina-Santillán NMS. New insights into the pathophysiology of non-alcoholic fatty liver disease. Annals of Hepatology. 2009;**8**(1):9-17

[21] Heyens LJM, Busschots D, Koek GH, Robaeys G, Francque S. Liver fibrosis in non-alcoholic fatty liver disease: From liver biopsy to non-invasive biomarkers in diagnosis and treatment. Frontier of Medicine;**8**:615978. DOI: 10.3389/fmed.2021.615978

[22] Chhimwal J, Vikram P, Yogendra P. Beverages and non-alcoholic fatty liver disease (NAFLD): Think before you drink. Clinical Nutrition. 2021;**40**:2508-2515

[23] Nseir W, Nassar F, Assy N. Soft drinks consumption and nonalcoholic fatty liver disease. World Journal of Gastroenterology. 2010;**16**(21):2579-2588. DOI: 10.3748/wjg.v16.i21.2579

[24] Hongwei C, Jue W, Zheng L, Christopher WKL, Ying X, Qibiao W, et al. Consumption of sugar-sweetened beverages has a dose-dependent effect on the risk of non-alcoholic fatty liver disease: An updated systematic review and dose-response meta-analysis. International Journal of Environmental Research Public Health. 2019;**16**:2192. DOI: 10.3390/ijerph16122192

[25] Ma J, Fox CS, Jacques PF, Speliotes EK, Hoffmann U, Smith CE, et al. Sugar-sweetened beverage, diet soda, and fatty liver disease in the Framingham Heart Study cohorts. Journal of Hepatology. Aug 2015;**63**(2):462-469. DOI: 10.1016/j.jhep.2015.03.032. Epub [5 Jun, 2015]

[26] Jomard A, Osto E. High density lipoproteins: Metabolism, function, and therapeutic potential. Frontiers in Cardiovascular Medicine. 2020;**7**:1-12

[27] Weaver JU. Practical Guide to Obesity Medicine. St. Louis Missouri: Elsevier; 2018. Available from: http://proxy.uqtr.ca/login.cgi?action=login&u=uqtr&db=sciencedir&ezurl=http://www.sciencedirect.com/science/book/9780323485593. Accessed [19 Oct, 2022]

[28] Karam I, Yang YJ, & Li JY. Atherosclerosis Hyperlipidemia Background and Progress. 2017

[29] Xenoulis PGSJ. Lipid metabolism and hyperlipidemia In dogs. The Veterinary Journal. 2010;**183**:12-21

[30] Wu MY, Li CJ, Hou MF, Chu PY. New insights into the role of inflammation in the Pathogenesis of Atherosclerosis. International Journal of Molecular Sciences. 2017;**18**(10):2034. Published 2017 Sep 22. DOI: 10.3390/ijms18102034

[31] Amit RM, David A, Joel NH. Chapter 4 - Genetics of Endocrinology. In: Shlomo M, Kenneth S, Polonsky P, Reed L, Henry M, Kronenberg W, editors. Textbook of Endocrinology (Thirteenth Edition). Elsevier; 2016. pp. 49-68. ISBN: 9780323297387. DOI: 10.1016/B978-0-323-29738-7.00004-6. Available from: https://www.sciencedirect.com/science/article/pii/B9780323297387000046

[32] Marques LR, Diniz TA, Antunes BM, et al. Reverse cholesterol transport: Molecular mechanisms and the non-medical approach to enhance HDL cholesterol. Frontiers in Physiology. 2018;**9**:1-11

[33] Trojak A, Waluś-Miarka M, Woźniakiewicz E, Małecki MT, Idzior-Waluś B. Nonalcoholic fatty liver disease is associated with low HDL cholesterol and coronary angioplasty in patients with type 2 diabetes. Medical Science Monitor. 2013;**19**:1167-1172. Published 2013 Dec 16. DOI: 10.12659/MSM.889649

[34] Catapano AL, Graham IG, Backer D, et al. 2016 ESC/EAS guidelines for the management of dyslipidaemias: The task force for the management of dyslipidaemias of the European Society of Cardiology (ESC) and European atherosclerosis society (EAS) developed with the special contribution of the Europe. Atherosclerosis. 2016;**253**:291-344

[35] Rosenson RS, Davidson MH, Hirsh BJ, Kathiresan S, Gaudet D. Genetics and causality of triglyceride-rich lipoproteins in atherosclerotic cardiovascular disease. Journal of the American College of Cardiology. 2014;**64**(23):2525-2540

Chapter 2

Hepatic Lipid Homeostasis in NAFLD

Shuo Zhang, Bing Ji, Changqing Yang and Li Yang

Abstract

Non-alcoholic fatty liver disease (NAFLD) is currently the most common liver disease, affecting 25% of world population. Hepatic steatosis has 60–90% prevalence among obese patients. It is also associated with multitude of detrimental effects and increased mortality. This narrative chapter investigates hepatic lipid homeostasis in NAFLD, focusing on the four molecular pathways of hepatic steatosis to lipid homeostasis in the liver. Hepatic steatosis is a consequence of lipid acquisition pathways exceeding lipid disposal pathways. In NAFLD, hepatic uptake of fatty acids and *de novo* lipogenesis surpass fatty acid oxidation and lipid export. The imbalance of the hepatic lipid may promote cellular damage by inducing oxidative stress in peroxisomes and cytochromes, especially with compromised mitochondrial function. Lipid export may even decrease with disease progression, sustaining the accumulation of lipids. NAFLD has a complex molecular mechanism regulating hepatic lipid homeostasis. Thus, as well as inter-individual differences, any intervention targeting one or more pathway is likely to have consequences on multiple cellular signaling pathways. We should be taken into careful consideration when developing future treatment options for NAFLD.

Keywords: non-alcoholic fatty liver disease, lipid metabolism, fatty acids uptake, *de novo* lipogenesis, triacylglycerol synthesis, lipophagy, very-low-density lipoprotein secretion

1. Introduction

Non-alcoholic fatty liver disease (NAFLD) is a spectrum of liver disorders defined by the presence of steatosis in more than 5% of hepatocytes with little or no alcohol consumption [1]. NAFLD is also associated with obesity, insulin resistance, type 2 diabetes mellitus (T2DM), hypertension, hyperlipidemia, and metabolic syndrome. Currently, NAFLD is increasing at approximately to be 25% in the general adult population [2–4] and 10% among children [5]. It encompasses six histological subtypes: simple liver steatosis, non-alcoholic steatohepatitis (NASH), non-alcoholic fibrosis, cirrhosis, hepatocellular carcinoma (HCC), and liver transplantation [6]. The global prevalence of NASH has been estimated to range from 3–5%. NAFLD is also associated with increased mortality, particularly due to cardiovascular disease, hepatocellular carcinoma, and liver-related events [7].

All of these complications of NASH can put significant health, economic, and patient-experience burdens to the patients and the society [8].

Hepatic steatosis is the hallmark of NAFLD, which also encompasses hepatic inflammation, hepatocyte damage, and even fibrosis, highlighting the potentially progressive nature of the disease. Although fibrosis also occurs in patients with steatosis alone, NASH has even higher rates of progression and overall mortality in NAFLD [9]. Additionally, hepatic steatosis is associated with metabolic dysfunctions, such as obesity status, insulin resistance, dyslipidemia, and cardiovascular disease [10].

The liver is an essential central regulator of lipid homeostasis organ, which is keeping the balance between lipid acquisition and disposal [11]. The liver acquires lipids through the uptake of circulating fatty acids (FAs) and *via de novo* lipogenesis (DNL) and be disposed of through fatty acid oxidation (FAO) in the mitochondria, peroxisomes, and cytochromes and through export as very low density lipoprotein (VLDL) particles. Lipid accumulation is the result of lipid acquisition pathways exceeding disposal pathways consequently. The disruption of one or more of these pathways may precipitate the retention of fat within the liver and the subsequent development of NAFLD. These processes are closely regulated by complex interactions between hormones, nuclear receptors, and transcription factors, keeping hepatic lipid homeostasis under tight control [12].

However, molecular mechanisms of hepatic lipid homeostasis in NAFLD are not fully elucidated. This chapter explores current insights into these four pathways and the molecular mechanisms regulating the pathological aggregation of NAFLD, discussing processes that may be instrumental in the development and progression of hepatic steatosis.

2. Hepatic FAs uptake

2.1 Plasma non-esterified FAs

There are several sources of FAs, including uptake from the blood and DNL, of which uptake from the blood is the major source of FAs for esterification into triacylglycerol (TG) in most conditions (**Figure 1**). The intracellular hydrolysis of TG in the adipose tissue is the largest contribution of FAs uptake from the blood [13], which is under the control of insulin. Insulin inhibits the activity of the two major lipolytic enzymes, including adipose triglyceride lipase (ATGL) and hormone-sensitive lipase. This dynamic process of FA uptake is upregulated during fasting conditions or insulin resistance, while downregulated during post-prandial period [14]. Although plasma concentration of FAs is often elevated in obesity and NAFLD, indicated the effect of insulin resistance, the relationship between insulin resistance and lipolysis is complex. It is identified that FAs release per kilogram fat mass is reduced in obesity, which might be associated with the downregulation of ATGL and hormone-sensitive lipase in adipose tissue [15]. In addition, the elevated postprandial FAs concentration could also be explained that insulin resistance reduces the insulin-mediated inhibition of adipose tissue TG hydrolysis in obesity [16]. Except for the condition of the body itself, the type and amount of dietary fat are also associated with subcutaneous adipose tissue lipolysis. Study found that high-fat diet could reduce the post-prandial suppression of adipose tissue lipolysis compared with moderate-fat diet [17]. Similarly, another study demonstrated that compared with unsaturated fat or free

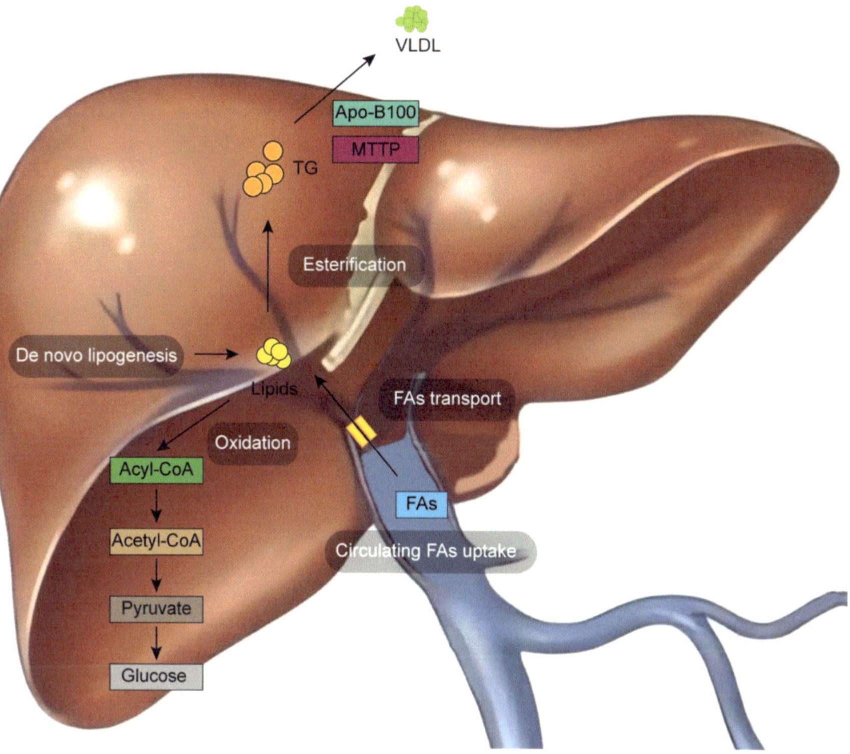

Figure 1.
Hepatic lipid metabolism. The homeostasis of intrahepatic lipid is governed by the four major pathways. Fatty acids (FAs), derived from blood circulation or de novo lipogenesis, can be stored in the form of lipid droplets (LDs). Conversely, FAs could be oxidized into acetyl-CoA as a substrate of ketone bodies, cholesterol, or glucose. FAs can also be esterified into triglyceride, which could form very low-density lipoprotein (VLDL) via apolipoprotein (Apo) B100 and microsomal TG transfer protein (MTTP) and further excreted from the liver.

sugar-enriched diet, diet enriched in saturated fat was associated with higher adipose tissue lipolysis [18].

Once flow to the hepatic vein, FAs are transported across the plasma membrane, mainly *via* transporter-mediated mechanisms, which is predominately mediated by fatty acid transport proteins (FATP), fatty acid translocase (FAT), also referred to as cluster of differentiation 36 (CD36), and caveolins located in the hepatocyte plasma membrane [19]. Studies found that the knockdown of FATP2 or FATP5, FATP isoforms primarily in the liver, reduces hepatocyte FAs uptake and further reverses steatosis [20, 21], indicating the FATP-mediated facilitation of steatosis. For CD36, it is regulated by peroxisome proliferator-activated receptor (PPAR) γ, pregnane X receptor, and liver X receptor (LXR) to facilitate long-chain FAs transportation. Studies identified that high-fat diet (HFD) upregulates mRNA and protein expression of CD36 and further aggravates hepatic steatosis, while liver-specific knockout of CD36 downregulates hepatic lipid levels and improves insulin resistance [22, 23]. CD36 is located in the hepatocyte plasma membrane in steatosis and NASH, while the expression of which is week in cytoplasm of hepatocytes in normal livers, which may indicate that the translocation of CD36 protein from cytoplasm to membrane could induce NAFLD progression (**Figure 2**) [24]. Caveolins are the third kind of transport-mediated protein, of which caveolin 1 is increased and mainly located in the centrilobular zone 3, the most severe part of steatosis in the liver with NAFLD. Study found that the upregulation of caveolin 1 might have clinical benefits in alleviating lipid accumulation in NAFLD [25, 26].

When uptake into cytoplasm, this hydrophobic FAs is binded with fatty acid-binding proteins (FABP) 1, the predominant isoform in the liver, to shuttle between different organelles. FABP1 could bind with cytotoxic-free FAs and promote its

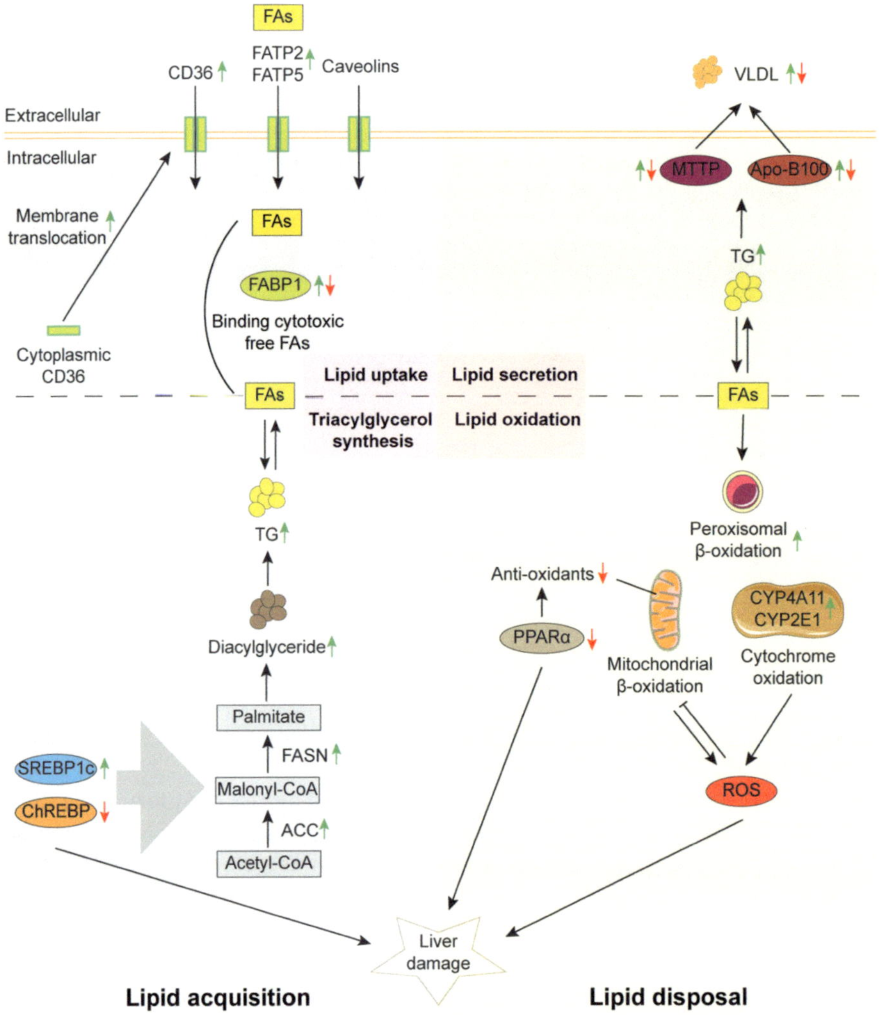

Figure 2.
Hepatic lipid metabolism in NAFLD. In NAFLD, cluster of differentiation 36 (CD36), fatty acid transport protein (FATP)-2 and -5 mediates uptake of circulating lipids increases. Fatty acid binding protein (FABP) 1 is increased in the early stage of disease and may decline with disease progression, which lead to lipotoxicity deterioration and disease progression. As for de novo lipogenesis, elevated sterol regulatory element-binding protein 1c (SREBP1c) and declined carbohydrate regulatory element-binding protein (ChREBP) enhance the downstream expression of acetyl-CoA carboxylase (ACC) and fatty acid synthase (FASN) in NAFLD. For lipid disposal, mitochondrial dysfunction may lead to increased generation of reactive oxygen species (ROS) and utilization of cytochrome- and peroxisome-mediated oxidation. Meanwhile, lipid export compensates for increased hepatic triglyceride levels in the early stage of disease. While the levels of microsomal triglyceride transfer protein (MTTP) and apolipoprotein B100 (ApoB100) may be decreased, therefore limiting very low density lipoprotein (VLDL) export and facilitating lipid accumulation in NASH. Green arrow: Increased expression. Red arrow: Decreased expression. PPAR, peroxisome proliferator-activated receptor.

oxidation and incorporation into TG, protecting the effect of lipotoxicity. In stage of steatosis, overexpression of FABP1 protein might enhance lipid flux to compensate lipotoxicity. While in the mid or late stage of NAFLD, presented as mild or advanced fibrosis, the level of FABP1 protein undergoes a series of decline, which leads to lipotoxicity deterioration and disease progression [27, 28].

2.2 Dietary chylomicrons

The contribution of dietary fat, in form of chylomicron remnants or chylomicron-derived spillover non-esterified fatty acids (NEFA), to liver fat accumulation depends on the amount and frequency of fat intake [29]. Chylomicron-derived TG is hydrolysed by lipoprotein lipase and mainly took up by adipose tissue, the rest of which is absorbed into the liver either by the LDL receptor (LDLR) or by the LDLR-related protein 1 (LRP1) [13, 30]. Once absorbed in the liver, chylomicron is hydrolysed by hepatic lysosomes to release FAs. In both obesity and NAFLD, hepatic expression of LDLR and LRP1 could be downregulated, which might be associated with the higher plasma concentrations of TG in these patients. Therefore, hepatic expression of LDLR and LRP1 participate in modulating the dyslipidemia and in preventing oxidized LDL-mediated liver injury.

3. FAs and triacylglycerol synthesis

3.1 *De novo* lipogenesis

Except uptake of circulating FAs, DNL enables liver to synthesize FAs by using non-lipid precursors (such as sugars and proteins) [31]. The production of acetyl-CoA initially provides the substrate required for DNL, which is converted to malonyl-CoA by acetyl-CoA carboxylase (ACC) and malonyl-CoA is then converted to palmitate by fatty acid synthase (FASN) [32]. The transcriptional regulation of DNL is mainly regulated by two transcription factors: sterol regulatory element-binding protein 1c (SREBP1c) and carbohydrate regulatory element-binding protein (ChREBP), which both stimulated by the activation of LXR and by nuclear translocation to activate target gene transcription [33, 34]. Studies identified that in NAFLD, SREBP1c expression is elevated, which is in agreement with hepatic TG levels, while SREBP1c knockout decreases the expression of lipogenic enzymes [33]. In addition, SREBP1c induces lipogenesis elevation and harmful lipid species accumulation, which might interfere with insulin signaling and therefore indirectly leads to the development of hepatic insulin resistance. When SREBP1c elevated, the expression of downstream targets ACC and FASN is accordingly increased in NAFLD [33, 35]. Although study demonstrated that knockout ACC1 could decrease hepatic lipid accumulation and inhibit DNL process, it may reactivity increase the expression of ACC2, which inhibits mitochondrial β-oxidation and leads to hepatic steatosis [36]. ACC1/2 inhibition could be a new option to improve hepatic steatosis in NAFLD [33]. As for another transcription factors, ChREBP participates in fructolysis, glycolysis, gluconeogenesis, and DNL pathways could mediate carbohydrate-associated DNL rather than induced by HFD [37]. Study found that high-fructose feeding could increase hepatocellular carbohydrate metabolites, expression of ChREBP target genes, and hepatic steatosis [38]. Inhibiting ChREBP expression could downregulate glucose-induced lipogenesis, which further reduces hepatic TG content and protect steatosis [39]. On the other hand, ChREBP knockout enhances cholesterol synthesis and its lipotoxicity and therefore induces hepatic steatosis, which may indicate the hepatoprotective effect of ChREBP [40].

Synthesized FAs may undergo a series of steps including desaturation, elongation, and esterification, and therefore ultimately being stored as a form of TG or exported in the form of VLDL particles. DNL was independently associated with intrahepatic TG levels [29]. Abnormally elevated DNL, occurred in NAFLD, could lead to the excessive production of saturated FAs (like palmitate), which induces steatohepatitis [41]. Besides, elevated DNL might also lead malonyl-CoA to inhibit the activity of carnitine palmitoyl transferase 1 (CPT1) suppressing hepatic FAs oxidation and increase ceramide synthesis from palmitoyl-CoA causing mitochondrial dysfunction, oxidative stress, and cell death. The above three effects may indirectly induce intrahepatic TG accumulation. Therefore, inadequate suppression of DNL is a feature of liver lipid accumulation in NAFLD.

3.2 Triacylglycerol synthesis

TG, synthesized by glycerol-3-phosphate acyltransferase (GPAT) or monoacylglycerol pathway *via* esterify fatty acyl-CoAs, is the major form of fat accumulated in the liver with NAFLD. The accumulation of TG in the liver, proved to be related to insulin resistance, is due to the abnormal balance between the hepatic DNL, TG synthesis, hepatic lipolysis, and lipid secretion. Although TG synthesis primarily occurs at the endoplasmic reticulum (ER), it can also occur at lipid droplets (LDs), mitochondria, and the nuclear envelope [42]. Several studies indicate that mitochondrial GPAT1 occupies 30–50% of the total GPAT activity in the liver, participating in hepatic steatosis [42]. The overexpression of GPAT1 in the rat liver was reported causing hepatic steatosis and insulin resistance in the absence of obesity or high-fat feeding [43]. In contrast, GPAT1 knockout mice showed remarkably lower hepatic TG concentrations and were prevented from hepatic steatosis and hepatic insulin resistance induced by HFD [44]. Inhibiting the activation of GPAT-1 might mitigate the progression of NAFLD.

4. Formation of hepatic LDs

LDs are specialized and dynamic cytosolic organelles, which mainly consist of a phospholipid monolayer with a core of neutral hydrophobic lipids (mostly TG and cholesterol ester, CE) [45]. As lipid storage reservoirs, LDs regulate the in- and out-flux of lipids, controlled by protein targeting process to prevent their accumulation and conversion to a toxic species. The most frequent proteins found in LDs are PLINs, especially PLIN2 and PLIN3 [21], which are involved in the formation of the LDs, during which enzymes including diacylglycerol O-acyltransferase 1, 2 (DGAT1, 2) and glycerol-3-phosphate acyltransferase 4 (GPAT4) localize around the droplet surface and further synthesize TG to store in the LDs. Researches hypothesized that LDs are formed when neutral lipids accumulate on the membranes of the ER, during which a lens is initially formed and then transforms into a budding LDs, and eventually buds off into the cytoplasm [46, 47].

The initial size of the LDs, fusion of cytoplasmic LDs, and *in situ* TG synthesis contributed to LDs growth. LDs form in the ER, where neutral lipids accumulate within the leaflet of the membrane bilayer. Once formed, small nascent LDs could be mediated by cell death-inducing DFFA-like effector proteins (CIDE), which lead to the fusion and formation of the large LD [45]. Under fasting or steatosis conditions, CIDEA and CIDEC could be induced to promote LD fusion [48, 49]. In addition to LDs fusion, there exists a potential phenomenon that lipid synthesis directly occurred on the surface of LDs or at newly formed LD-ER membrane bridges, which may also result in LDs expansion. Besides, TG synthesis such as acyl-CoA synthetases as well as the acyltransferases GPAT4 and DGAT2 could expand LD monolayer membrane by inducing excessive TG into the LD core [47, 50]. Once reaching critical concentration, LDs are budded and excreted into the cytoplasm, referred to as a phase separation of the bilayer, and continue to grow the size of LDs. As for LDs budding, *in vitro* studies recently found that several factors could drive the differences in the phospholipid composition between the two leaflets, result in tension asymmetry, which therefore favor budding toward the side with lower monolayer tension [51]. Fat storage-inducing transmembrane protein 2 (FIT2), an integral endoplasmic reticulum membrane protein with lipid-phosphate phosphatase activity, is required for correct budding of nascent LDs, which might promote LDs budding by inducing membrane asymmetries between the ER bilayers. Besides, other factors, including the asymmetric insertion of proteins at the bilayer, the asymmetric acting of lipid-modifying enzymes on leaflets of the bilayer, or an asymmetric refill of newly synthesized phospholipids, may also lead to the asymmetric surface tension of the leaflets.

5. Lipid mobilization and degradation

5.1 Lipolysis

In hepatocytes, lipolysis and lipophagy together participate in lipids mobilization, which are further degraded by β-oxidation. The lipolysis of LDs involves the coordinated response of surface proteins and corresponding enzymes. Intracellular lipolysis can be divided into neutral and acid lipolysis, depending on the pH value and the corresponding subcellular location.

Neutral lipolysis of TG occurs in the cytoplasm with neutral pH, during which the TG and CE stored in LDs are directly degraded by the consecutive action of the three neutral lipases, including patatin-like phospholipase domain-containing protein 2 (PNPLA2), LIPE/HSL (lipase E, hormone-sensitive type), and monoglyceride lipase (MGL) [52]. Studies found that ATGL encoded by the patatin-like phospholipase domain-containing protein 2 (PNPLA2) gene may participate in NAFLD, of which ATGL knockout leads to LDs accumulation, while overexpression of ATGL could alleviate hepatic steatosis and increase FAs oxidation [53, 54]. Recent study identified that despite enhancing hepatic steatosis, ATGL/PNPLA2 deficiency may decrease hepatic lipolysis and increase PPARδ, which protects hepatocyte from inflammation and ER stress [55]. HSL was considered a rate-limiting enzyme for TG hydrolysis. HSL deficiency, characterized by relatively mild forms of dyslipidemia and hepatic steatosis, manifests in a more benign phenotype than does ATGL deficiency [56]. Besides, HSL could bind to CHREBP to prevent its translocation into the nucleus and downregulate its transcriptional activity of CHREBP [57]. MGL is the rate-limiting enzyme of monoacylglycerol (MG) degradation that derives from phospholipids or TG. Study found that MGL deficiency in mice leads to MG accumulation, minor changes of plasma VLDL metabolism, and a moderate protection from diet-induced hepatic steatosis [58]. Besides, MGL inhibition could attenuate LPS-induced inflammation in liver [59]. Hypoxia training may induce MGL expression and ameliorate hepatic steatosis [60].

Acid lipolysis, mediated by lipases such as the lipase A and lysosomal acid (LIPA/LAL), occurs in acidic pH inside lysosome, which could hydrolyze lipids delivered into lysosomes through receptor-mediated endocytosis of lipoproteins and lipophagy and further produce free cholesterol and FAs [61]. The reduction of LAL activity causes intra-lysosomal CE accumulation and lowers free cholesterol in cytosol, which could induce transcription factor promoting lipogenesis and synthesis of cholesterol and of VLDL [62]. Clinical study has demonstrated that blood LAL levels at different stages of NAFLD evolution are gradually declined [63]. In addition, impaired LAL activity appears specific to NAFLD in the context of liver disease.

5.2 Lipophagy

In addition to the actions of lipolysis, lipophagy plays a role in lipid mobilization and degradation in hepatocytes (**Figure 3**). Lipophagy could act as the downstream of lipolysis, since large LDs could produce small LDs by re-esterification *via* ATGL that can subsequently be targeted by lipophagy [64]. Depending on the manner of LDs transportation into lysosomes and vacuoles, lipophagy could be divided into macro- and microautophagy [52]. Macrolipophagy involves the autophagosome-mediated LDs sequestration and their subsequent delivery to lysosomes/vacuole for degradation by lysosomal acid lipase, while microlipophagy is the process through which LDs and lysosomes take place direct physical interaction and transferation of lipids [65]. Inhibition of lipophagy could lead to TG and LDs accumulation *in vitro* and *in vivo*, a decrease in TG breakdown and a colocalization between TG components and TG or LDs proteins [52, 66]. Dysregulation of lipophagy may induce hepatic lipid accumulation and therefore lead to NAFLD.

Increasing evidence supports the ATGL-mediated interplay between lipolysis and lipophagy for different size of LDs [66]. Lysosomal inhibition has been shown to lead to the accumulation of small LDs within autophagosomes, which demonstrated that macrolipophagy primarily targets small LDs. Study identifies that ATGL participates in neutral lipolysis to decrease the size of large LDs and create small newly LDs, accessible for sequestration of macrolipophagy, *via* FAs re-esterification [67]. ATGL may also activate sirtuin 1 (SIRT1) to promote LDs degradation by macrolipophagy [68]. Besides, ER stress inhibits macrolipophagy by downregulating the fusion between the autophagosome and the lysosome, which could lead to accumulation of ubiquitinated proteins and LDs that in turn increase ER stress and reactive oxygen species (ROS) production. HFD-induced mice liver may lead to the altered lipid composition of autophagosomes and/or lysosomes, which in turn affects their fusion and impaired lipophagy [69]. In addition, excess nutrient supply may alter the upstream kinase pathways of lipophagy and impair its function. The MAP3K5/ASK1 (mitogen-activated protein kinase 5), a regulator of the MAPK signaling cascades, negatively correlates with hepatic lipids accumulation and NASH scores, and positively correlates with TG level, suggesting its macroautophagy-related protective role [70], on the other hand MAP3K5 inhibition is reported to reduce hepatic lipid accumulation and inflammation [71]. The effect of MAP3K5 on NAFLD may need to be further investigated.

In some cases, lysosomes can directly engulf one relatively large LD, supporting the existence of microlipophagy in hepatocytes. Compared with macroautophagy, microlipophagy may be a more efficient pathway for small LDs degradation without

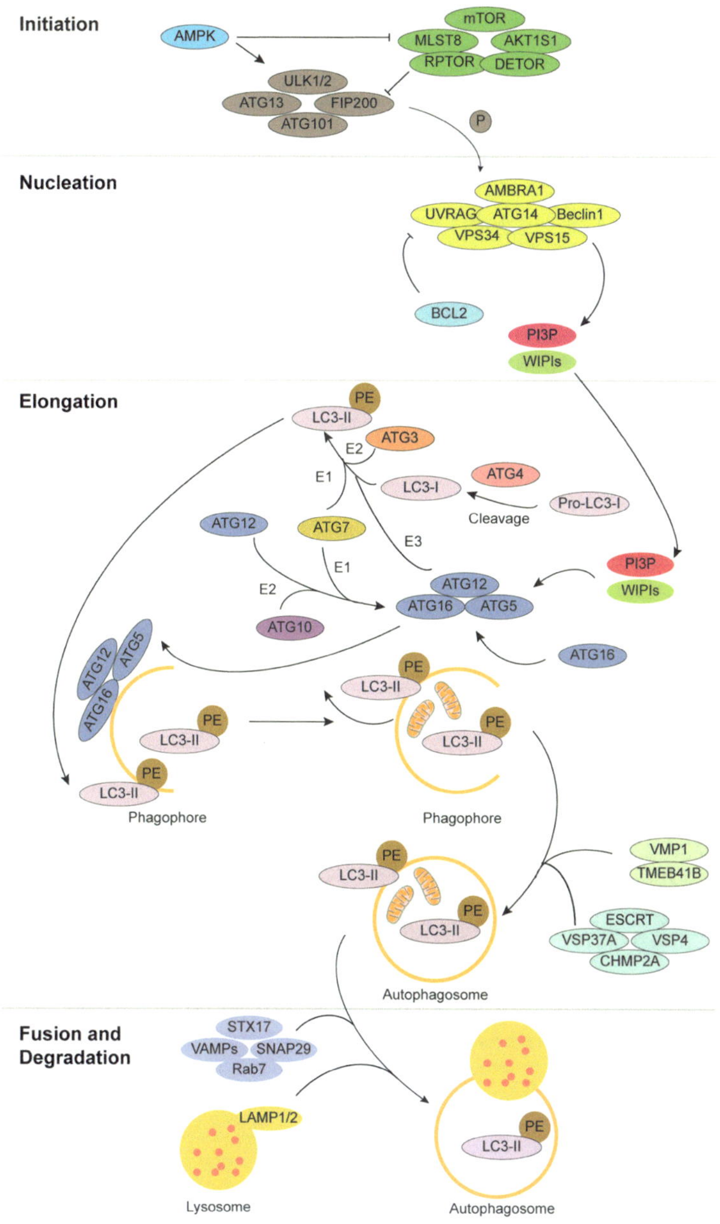

Figure 3.
A scheme of the lipophagy process. Lipophagy caused by nutrient deficiency can be divided into five main stages: (1) initiation, (2) nucleation, (3) extension, (4) fusion, and (5) degradation. The increase of cAMP/ATP ratio can activate AMPK, which inhibits mTORC1 and activates ULK1/2 through direct or indirect phosphorylation. The formed ULK1/2-ATG13-ATG101-focal adhesion kinase family interacting protein of 200 KD (FIP200) complex activates Beclin 1 and interacts with UVRAG, autophagy, and Beclin 1 regulator 1 (AMBRA1), VPS34 phosphoinositide-3-kinase regulatory subunit 4 (PI3KR4, such as VPS15) binds to form phosphatidylinositol 3-phosphate (PI3P) and connects with WD repeat protein interacting with phosphoinositides (WIPIs) to participate in the nucleation and elongation. In the elongation stage, ATG7 and ATG10 ligases connect ATG12 with ATG5 and combine with polyprotein ATG16 to form a complex by promoting ATG7 (E1) and ATG10 (E2). Pro-LC3-I is combined with phosphatidylethanolamine (PE) through ATG4, ATG7, and ATG3 to form LC3-II. LC3-II binds to the expanding autophagy membrane, recruits transporters such as P62/SQSTM1, and selects and wraps components such as cytoplasm or organelles in cells. Closed autophagosomes fuse with lysosomes to produce autophagy lysosomes, causing lumen acidification, hydrolase activation, and content degradation.

using autophagosomes [52]. Studies have reported that the process of microlipophagy needs the core TG machinery [72, 73], while others demonstrate that microlipophagy does not require core TG proteins [74]. At present, there is insufficient research on the correlation between microlipophagy and NAFLD, and studies are needed to unveil its precise mechanism.

5.3 Hepatic FAs oxidation

Hepatic FAs oxidation (FAO), commonly induced by low-circulating glucose concentrations, occurs mainly in the mitochondria to provide energy, which is controlled by PPARα [75]. FAs are transported into the mitochondria *via* CPT1 situated in the outer mitochondrial membrane and preferably metabolized *via* peroxisomal β-oxidation.

The action of PPARα is upregulated by FAs and glucagon and suppressed by insulin. PPARα activation could induce the transcription of FAO-related genes in the mitochondria, peroxisomes, and cytochromes, which therefore reduces the level of hepatic lipids [76]. PPARα knockout could lead to hepatic steatosis in mice, emphasizing the critical role of PPARα in promoting FAO and preventing hepatic lipid accumulation [77]. However, studies of FAO are conflicting in patients with NAFLD. Increased FAO might be a compensatory response in NAFLD to reduce the lipids accumulation and lipotoxicity, which could also produce ROS to induce oxidative stress. Compared to patients with less severe steatosis or non-steatotic controls, the expression of β-oxidation-related genes was higher in patients with more severe steatosis [78]. Combination of stable isotope-labeled tracers identified that fasting mitochondrial oxidation was twice as high in patients with NAFLD than in those without NAFLD [79]. FAs oxidation and its oxidative damage to mitochondrial DNA occur in NAFLD, which could further impair mitochondrial function, resulting in a vicious cycle and alteration of mitochondrial ultrastructure [79]. Study found that FAO and the rate-limiting enzyme in β-oxidation of hepatic mitochondrial were reduced in definite NASH compared with no disease controls [80]. In addition, FAs-metabolizing enzyme located in the cytochromes such as CYP2E1 and CYP4A11 elevates in the context of NAFLD. Increased FAO in cytochromes may induce excess accumulation of ROS and exacerbation of hepatic oxidative stress, which could lead to hepatic steatosis.

6. Hepatic FAs secretion

Except FAO, non-oxidized FAs in the liver could be esterified into TG and then used for VLDL secretion. During this time, circulating lipids could undergo a series of process, including internalization, procession and incorporation into TG, CE and membrane lipids, and TG secretion, by which hydrophobic FAs are released into the blood stream as the form of VLDL [81]. VLDL is initially formed with the transfer of a apolipoprotein B100 (ApoB100) from the rough to the smooth ER, in which a primordial VLDL particle is form by the addition of TG via microsomal TG transfer protein (MTTP). Then, the nascent VLDL particle is transferred to the Golgi apparatus and further forms a mature VLDL particle [82].

The link has been established between increased VLDL secretion and metabolic diseases [81, 82]. Although studies found that the greater availability of TG and higher MTTP activity could promote VLDL particle production and plasma TG concentrations [82, 83], there do not exist a definite positive correlation between plasma TG concentrations and the hepatic steatosis. In response to excess hepatic fat, NAFLD patients actually secrete more VLDL-TG than do subjects without NAFLD. ApoB100 and MTTP are associated with VLDL secretion, and serve as key components in hepatic VLDL secretion and in maintaining hepatic lipid homeostasis. The transcription of MTTP could be upregulated by PPARα and its expression parallels with ApoB100 secretion, while insulin could reduce hepatic lipid secretion by inducing ApoB100 degradation and suppressing MTTP synthesis, which downregulates both ApoB100 and MTTP [83, 84]. In normal liver, high level of insulin levels during post-prandial state facilitates the mobilization of dietary lipids rather than hepatic VLDL, while the selective hepatic insulin resistance in NAFLD may induce insulin to stimulate DNL without inhibiting VLDL production, indirectly increasing the secretion of VLDL. Although VLDL particles overproduction has been reported in patients with NAFLD, ApoB100 secretion is unchanged. Further study demonstrated that VLDL particles secreted as a more TG-rich and larger form than those in normal people [85]. Notably, while intrahepatic lipid accumulation increases VLDL-TG secretion, when hepatic fat content exceeded 10%, the capacity of VLDL-TG secretion is unable to compensate the lipid metabolic homeostasis. Besides, compared to no disease controls, NAFLD patients with more advanced steatosis had lower MTTP levels, which indicate that lipids accumulation may impair lipid secretion [81].

The association between dietary structure and VLDL secretion has been identified in several studies, which suggest the more significant effect of sugar than that of fat and carbohydrate on VLDL secretion. A study compared the influence of sugar-enriched diet and less sugar diet, which found that the former could significantly increase the VLDL1-TG production rate in patients with or without NAFLD [86], while the VLDL2 production rate increased only after the high sugar diet in NAFLD [86]. While for dietary fat, study found that the level of monounsaturated FAs in the diet may not affect the production of VLDL1 and VLDL2 in patients with mild hypercholesterolemia [87]. Moreover, study demonstrated that although high-carbohydrate diet could induce higher VLDL-TG concentrations and a lower VLDL-TG uptake than control diet in normal or hypertriglyceridemia individuals, two groups did not have different responses [88].

7. Diagnosis and management of NAFLD

Liver biopsy is the gold standard to diagnose NAFLD. However, this procedure is invasive, expensive, and time-consuming, which limits its clinical application [89, 90]. MRI is highly sensitive and offers the possibility to quantitate fat tissue, which might be limited by high costs. Elastography could determine the elastic properties of liver; however, the thickness of peripheral tissue contributes as limiting factor. As for serological method, although ALT shows a low specificity for NAFLD, it still be the most common diagnostic biomarker. Besides, cytokeratin-18 (CK18) could be used to diagnose NASH. Lipidomics serves as a new method and could utilize the specific signature of various lipids to identify NAFLD, of which studies found that lysophospholipids (LPLs), TG, bis-(monoacylglycerol)-phosphate (BMP), 5-, 8-, 11-hydroxyeicosatetraenoic acids (5-,8-,11-HETEs), 9-,13-hydroxyoctadecadienoic acids (9-,13-HODEs), and short- and medium-chain TG are elevated, while phosphoinositols (PI), phosphatidylethanolamines (PE), and phosphatidylcholines (PC) are reduced [91–94].

Decreasing the synthesis and/or increasing the disposal of intrahepatic FAs has been suggested to attenuate the risk of NAFLD. Lifestyle interventions composing of diet, exercise, and weight loss remain the optimal therapeutic strategy, of which general caloric restriction is one of the most effective ways to reduce liver FAs uptake. While, compared with general caloric restriction, studies indicated the additional metabolic benefits of intermittent fasting, including a reduction of hepatic steatosis, inflammation and PKCε activation, and increased insulin sensitivity [95, 96]. A meta-analysis found that people lose at least 5% of body weight could improve hepatic steatosis and lose at least 7% of body weight could improve NASH [97]. Therefore, caloric restriction and loss weight are the important measures to relieve NAFLD.

For patients failed to achieve lifestyle modification, pharmacological medication may be needed to reduce FAs accumulation. Several studies target to inhibit either ACC or DGAT2, which could reduce DNL and therefore lower the concentration of TG [98, 99]. Meanwhile, pathways associated with insulin resistance have been demonstrated as a therapeutic target of NAFLD, including bile acid-based insulin sensitization, peroxisome proliferator-activator receptors, FGF21, and metformin. Obeticholic acid (OCA), a selective farnesoid X receptor (FXR) agonist, is the first synthetic bile acid for the treatment of NASH that showed the potential anti-inflammatory and anti-fibrotic effects in the liver [100]. Thiazolidinedione, a selective ligand of the PPARs, seems to decrease IHTAG content [101]. Additionally, saroglitazar was demonstrated lowering steatosis and ALT in mouse with NASH [102]. Moreover, supplementation with n-3 polyunsaturated fatty acid (PUFA) could also reduce the concentration of TG [103].

8. Conclusion

NAFLD is the pathological state co-mediated by several stages, involving hepatic FAs uptake, FAs and TG synthesis, hepatic LDs formation, lipid mobilization and degradation, and FAs secretion. Current studies suggest that dietary structure and genetic variants are likely to alter metabolic pathways that lead to the imbalance of hepatic FAs uptake and utilization. There exist complex mechanisms to maintain hepatic lipid homeostasis and prevent chronic lipid overload, which may indicate any intervention on lipid metabolic pathway lead to significant consequences on lipid homeostasis. Therefore, the effect of individual differences on disease occurrence and prognosis need to be awarded in further research and treatment of NAFLD.

Conflict of interest

The authors declare no conflict of interest.

Author details

Shuo Zhang†, Bing Ji†, Changqing Yang† and Li Yang*
Department of Gastroenterology and Hepatology, Shanghai Tongji Hospital, School of Medicine, Tongji University, Shanghai, China

*Address all correspondence to: liyang19732003@tongji.edu.cn

† These authors contributed equally to this work.

References

[1] Sanyal AJ, Brunt EM, Kleiner DE, et al. Endpoints and clinical trial design for nonalcoholic steatohepatitis. Hepatology. 2011;**54**(1):344-353. DOI: 10.1002/hep.24376

[2] Vernon G, Baranova A, Younossi ZM. Systematic review: The epidemiology and natural history of non-alcoholic fatty liver disease and non-alcoholic steatohepatitis in adults. Alimentary Pharmacology & Therapeutics. 2011;**34**(3):274-285. DOI: 10.1111/j.1365-2036.2011.04724.x

[3] Younossi Z, Anstee QM, Marietti M, et al. Global burden of NAFLD and NASH: Trends, predictions, risk factors and prevention. Nature Reviews. Gastroenterology & Hepatology. 2018;**15**(1):11-20. DOI: 10.1038/nrgastro.2017.109

[4] Fan JG, Kim SU, Wong VW. New trends on obesity and NAFLD in Asia. Journal of Hepatology. 2017;**67**(4):862-873. DOI: 10.1016/j.jhep.2017.06.003

[5] Schwimmer JB, Deutsch R, Kahen T, et al. Prevalence of fatty liver in children and adolescents. Pediatrics. 2006;**118**(4):1388-1393. DOI: 10.1542/peds.2006-1212

[6] Younossi Z, Tacke F, Arrese M, et al. Global perspectives on nonalcoholic fatty liver disease and nonalcoholic steatohepatitis. Hepatology. 2019;**69**(6):2672-2682. DOI: 10.1002/hep.30251

[7] Adams LA, Anstee QM, Tilg H, et al. Non-alcoholic fatty liver disease and its relationship with cardiovascular disease and other extrahepatic diseases. Gut. 2017;**66**(6):1138-1153. DOI: 10.1136/gutjnl-2017-313884

[8] Younossi ZM, Koenig AB, Abdelatif D, et al. Global epidemiology of nonalcoholic fatty liver disease—Meta-analytic assessment of prevalence, incidence, and outcomes. Hepatology. 2016;**64**(1):73-84. DOI: 10.1002/hep.28431

[9] Singh S, Allen AM, Wang Z, et al. Fibrosis progression in nonalcoholic fatty liver vs nonalcoholic steatohepatitis: A systematic review and meta-analysis of paired-biopsy studies. Clinical Gastroenterology and Hepatology. 2015;**13**(4):643-654. DOI: 10.1016/j.cgh.2014.04.014

[10] Fabbrini E, Magkos F. Hepatic steatosis as a marker of metabolic dysfunction. Nutrients. 2015;7(6):4995-5019. DOI: 10.3390/nu7064995

[11] Nguyen P, Leray V, Diez M, et al. Liver lipid metabolism. Journal of Animal Physiology and Animal Nutrition (Berlin). 2008;**92**(3):272-283. DOI: 10.1111/j.1439-0396.2007.00752.x

[12] Bechmann LP, Hannivoort RA, Gerken G, et al. The interaction of hepatic lipid and glucose metabolism in liver diseases. Journal of Hepatology. 2012;**56**(4):952-964. DOI: 10.1016/j.jhep.2011.08.025

[13] Piché ME, Parry SA, Karpe F, et al. Chylomicron-derived fatty acid spillover in adipose tissue: A signature of metabolic health? The Journal of Clinical Endocrinology and Metabolism. 2018;**103**(1):25-34. DOI: 10.1210/jc.2017-01517

[14] Ruge T, Hodson L, Cheeseman J, et al. Fasted to fed trafficking of fatty acids in human adipose tissue reveals a novel regulatory step for enhanced

fat storage. The Journal of Clinical Endocrinology and Metabolism. 2009;**94**(5):1781-1788. DOI: 10.1210/jc.2008-2090

[15] Karpe F, Dickmann JR, Frayn KN. Fatty acids, obesity, and insulin resistance: Time for a reevaluation. Diabetes. 2011;**60**(10):2441-2449. DOI: 10.2337/db11-0425

[16] McQuaid SE, Hodson L, Neville MJ, et al. Downregulation of adipose tissue fatty acid trafficking in obesity: A driver for ectopic fat deposition? Diabetes. 2011;**60**(1):47-55. DOI: 10.2337/db10-0867

[17] Howe HR 3rd, Heidal K, Choi MD, et al. Increased adipose tissue lipolysis after a 2-week high-fat diet in sedentary overweight/obese men. Metabolism. 2011;**60**(7):976-981. DOI: 10.1016/j.metabol.2010.09.007

[18] Luukkonen PK, Sädevirta S, Zhou Y, et al. Saturated fat is more metabolically harmful for the human liver than unsaturated fat or simple sugars. Diabetes Care. 2018;**41**(8):1732-1739. DOI: 10.2337/dc18-0071

[19] Koo SH. Nonalcoholic fatty liver disease: Molecular mechanisms for the hepatic steatosis. Clinical and Molecular Hepatology. 2013;**19**(3):210-215. DOI: 10.3350/cmh.2013.19.3.210

[20] Falcon A, Doege H, Fluitt A, et al. FATP2 is a hepatic fatty acid transporter and peroxisomal very long-chain acyl-CoA synthetase. American Journal of Physiology. Endocrinology and Metabolism. 2010;**299**(3):E384-E393. DOI: 10.1152/ajpendo.00226.2010

[21] Doege H, Baillie RA, Ortegon AM, et al. Targeted deletion of FATP5 reveals multiple functions in liver metabolism: Alterations in hepatic lipid homeostasis. Gastroenterology. 2006;**130**(4):1245-1258. DOI: 10.1053/j.gastro.2006.02.006

[22] Wilson CG, Tran JL, Erion DM, et al. Hepatocyte-specific disruption of CD36 attenuates fatty liver and improves insulin sensitivity in HFD-fed mice. Endocrinology. 2016;**157**(2):570-585. DOI: 10.1210/en.2015-1866

[23] Koonen DP, Jacobs RL, Febbraio M, et al. Increased hepatic CD36 expression contributes to dyslipidemia associated with diet-induced obesity. Diabetes. 2007;**56**(12):2863-2871. DOI: 10.2337/db07-0907

[24] Glatz JFC, Luiken JJFP. Dynamic role of the transmembrane glycoprotein CD36 (SR-B2) in cellular fatty acid uptake and utilization. Journal of Lipid Research. 2018;**59**(7):1084-1093. DOI: 10.1194/jlr.R082933

[25] Wang J, Jiang W, Xin J, et al. Caveolin-1 alleviates acetaminophen-induced fat accumulation in non-alcoholic fatty liver disease by enhancing hepatic antioxidant ability via activating AMPK pathway. Frontiers in Pharmacology. 2021;**12**:717276. DOI: 10.3389/fphar.2021.717276

[26] Xue W, Wang J, Jiang W, et al. Caveolin-1 alleviates lipid accumulation in NAFLD associated with promoting autophagy by inhibiting the Akt/mTOR pathway. European Journal of Pharmacology. 2020;**871**:172910. DOI: 10.1016/j.ejphar.2020.172910

[27] Charlton M, Viker K, Krishnan A, et al. Differential expression of lumican and fatty acid binding protein-1: New insights into the histologic spectrum of nonalcoholic fatty liver disease. Hepatology. 2009;**49**(4):1375-1384. DOI: 10.1002/hep.22927

[28] Lu YC, Chang CC, Wang CP, et al. Circulating fatty acid-binding protein 1 (FABP1) and nonalcoholic fatty liver disease in patients with type 2 diabetes mellitus. International Journal of Medical Sciences. 2020;**17**(2):182-190. DOI: 10.7150/ijms.40417

[29] Hodson L. Hepatic fatty acid synthesis and partitioning: The effect of metabolic and nutritional state. The Proceedings of the Nutrition Society. 2019;**78**(1):126-134. DOI: 10.1017/S0029665118002653

[30] Babin PJ, Gibbons GF. The evolution of plasma cholesterol: Direct utility or a "spandrel" of hepatic lipid metabolism? Progress in Lipid Research. 2009;**48**(2):73-91. DOI: 10.1016/j.plipres.2008.11.002

[31] Suppli MP, Rigbolt KTG, Veidal SS, et al. Hepatic transcriptome signatures in patients with varying degrees of nonalcoholic fatty liver disease compared with healthy normal-weight individuals. American Journal of Physiology. Gastrointestinal and Liver Physiology. 2019;**316**(4):G462-G472. DOI: 10.1152/ajpgi.00358.2018

[32] Wang Y, Yu W, Li S, et al. Acetyl-CoA carboxylases and diseases. Front. Oncologia. 2022;**12**:836058. DOI: 10.3389/fonc.2022.836058

[33] Wang Y, Viscarra J, Kim SJ, et al. Transcriptional regulation of hepatic lipogenesis. Nature Reviews. Molecular Cell Biology. 2015;**16**(11):678-689. DOI: 10.1038/nrm4074

[34] Linden AG, Li S, Choi HY, et al. Interplay between ChREBP and SREBP-1c coordinates postprandial glycolysis and lipogenesis in livers of mice. Journal of Lipid Research. 2018;**59**(3):475-487. DOI: 10.1194/jlr.M081836

[35] Xie Z, Li H, Wang K, et al. Analysis of transcriptome and metabolome profiles alterations in fatty liver induced by high-fat diet in rat. Metabolism. 2010;**59**(4):554-560. DOI: 10.1016/j.metabol.2009.08.022

[36] Mao J, DeMayo FJ, Li H, et al. Liver-specific deletion of acetyl-CoA carboxylase 1 reduces hepatic triglyceride accumulation without affecting glucose homeostasis. Proceedings of the National Academy of Sciences of the United States of America. 2006;**103**(22):8552-8557. DOI: 10.1073/pnas.0603115103

[37] Ter Horst KW, Serlie MJ. Fructose consumption, lipogenesis, and non-alcoholic fatty liver disease. Nutrients. 2017;**9**(9):981. DOI: 10.3390/nu9090981

[38] Kim MS, Krawczyk SA, Doridot L, et al. ChREBP regulates fructose-induced glucose production independently of insulin signaling. The Journal of Clinical Investigation. 2016;**126**(11):4372-4386. DOI: 10.1172/JCI81993

[39] Dentin R, Benhamed F, Hainault I, et al. Liver-specific inhibition of ChREBP improves hepatic steatosis and insulin resistance in ob/ob mice. Diabetes. 2006;**55**(8):2159-2170. DOI: 10.2337/db06-0200

[40] Zhang D, Tong X, VanDommelen K, et al. Lipogenic transcription factor ChREBP mediates fructose-induced metabolic adaptations to prevent hepatotoxicity. The Journal of Clinical Investigation. 2017;**127**(7):2855-2867. DOI: 10.1172/JCI89934

[41] Alsabeeh N, Chausse B, Kakimoto PA, et al. Cell culture models of fatty acid overload: Problems and solutions. Biochimica et Biophysica Acta—Molecular and Cell Biology of Lipids. 2018;**1863**(2):143-151. DOI: 10.1016/j.bbalip.2017.11.006

[42] Wang H, Airola MV, Reue K. How lipid droplets "TAG" along: Glycerolipid synthetic enzymes and lipid storage. Biochimica et Biophysica Acta—Molecular and Cell Biology of Lipids. 2017;**1862**(10 Pt B):1131-1145. DOI: 10.1016/j.bbalip.2017.06.010

[43] Nagle CA, An J, Shiota M, et al. Hepatic overexpression of glycerol-sn-3-phosphate acyltransferase 1 in rats causes insulin resistance. The Journal of Biological Chemistry. 2007;**282**(20):14807-14815. DOI: 10.1074/jbc.M611550200

[44] Neschen S, Morino K, Hammond LE, et al. Prevention of hepatic steatosis and hepatic insulin resistance in mitochondrial acyl-CoA: Glycerol-sn-3-phosphate acyltransferase 1 knockout mice. Cell Metabolism. 2005;**2**(1):55-65. DOI: 10.1016/j.cmet.2005.06.006

[45] Gluchowski NL, Becuwe M, Walther TC, et al. Lipid droplets and liver disease: From basic biology to clinical implications. Nature Reviews. Gastroenterology & Hepatology. 2017;**14**(6):343-355. DOI: 10.1038/nrgastro.2017.32

[46] Walther TC, Chung J, Farese RV Jr. Lipid droplet biogenesis. Annual Review of Cell and Developmental Biology. 2017;**33**:491-510. DOI: 10.1146/annurev-cellbio-100616-060608

[47] Gao M, Huang X, Song BL, et al. The biogenesis of lipid droplets: Lipids take center stage. Progress in Lipid Research. 2019;**75**:100989

[48] Xu W, Wu L, Yu M, et al. Differential roles of cell death-inducing DNA fragmentation factor-α-like effector (CIDE) proteins in promoting lipid droplet fusion and growth in subpopulations of hepatocytes. Journal of Biological Chemistry. 2016;**291**(9):4282-4293

[49] Langhi C, Baldán Á. CIDEC/FSP27 is regulated by peroxisome proliferator-activated receptor alpha and plays a critical role in fasting- and diet-induced hepatosteatosis. Hepatology. 2015;**61**(4):1227-1238

[50] Wilfling F, Wang H, Haas JT, et al. Triacylglycerol synthesis enzymes mediate lipid droplet growth by relocalizing from the ER to lipid droplets. Developmental Cell. 2013;**24**(4):384-399

[51] Chorlay A, Thiam AR. An asymmetry in monolayer tension regulates lipid droplet budding direction. Biophysical Journal. 2018;**114**(3):631-640. DOI: 10.1016/j.bpj.2017.12.014

[52] Filali-Mouncef Y, Hunter C, Roccio F, et al. The ménage à trois of autophagy, lipid droplets and liver disease. Autophagy. 2022;**18**(1):50-72. DOI: 10.1080/15548627.2021.1895658

[53] Wu JW, Wang SP, Alvarez F, et al. Deficiency of liver adipose triglyceride lipase in mice causes progressive hepatic steatosis. Hepatology. 2011;**54**(1):122-132. DOI: 10.1002/hep.24338

[54] Turpin SM, Hoy AJ, Brown RD, et al. Adipose triacylglycerol lipase is a major regulator of hepatic lipid metabolism but not insulin sensitivity in mice. Diabetologia. 2011;**54**(1):146-156. DOI: 10.1007/s00125-010-1895-5

[55] Fuchs CD, Radun R, Dixon ED, et al. Hepatocyte-specific deletion of adipose triglyceride lipase (adipose triglyceride lipase/patatin-like phospholipase domain containing 2) ameliorates dietary induced steatohepatitis in mice. Hepatology. 2022;**75**(1):125-139. DOI: 10.1002/hep.32112

[56] Grabner GF, Xie H, Schweiger M, et al. Lipolysis: Cellular mechanisms for lipid mobilization from fat stores. Nature Metabolism. 2021;**3**(11):1445-1465. DOI: 10.1038/s42255-021-00493-6

[57] Morigny P, Houssier M, Mairal A, et al. Interaction between hormone-sensitive lipase and ChREBP in fat cells controls insulin sensitivity. Nature Metabolism. 2019;**1**(1):133-146. DOI: 10.1038/s42255-018-0007-6

[58] Tardelli M, Bruschi FV, Claudel T, et al. Lack of monoacylglycerol lipase prevents hepatic steatosis by favoring lipid storage in adipose tissue and intestinal malabsorption. Journal of Lipid Research. 2019;**60**(7):1284-1292. DOI: 10.1194/jlr.M093369

[59] Cao Z, Mulvihill MM, Mukhopadhyay P, et al. Monoacylglycerol lipase controls endocannabinoid and eicosanoid signaling and hepatic injury in mice. Gastroenterology. 2013;**144**(4):808-817.e15. DOI: 10.1053/j.gastro.2012.12.028

[60] Yang Q, Sun S, Liu W, et al. Hypoxia training improves hepatic steatosis partly by downregulation of CB1 receptor in obese mice. Biochemical and Biophysical Research Communications. 2020;**525**(3):639-645. DOI: 10.1016/j.bbrc.2020.02.134

[61] Zechner R, Madeo F, Kratky D. Cytosolic lipolysis and lipophagy: Two sides of the same coin. Nature Reviews. Molecular Cell Biology. 2017;**18**(11):671-684. DOI: 10.1038/nrm.2017.76

[62] Baratta F, Pastori D, Ferro D, et al. Reduced lysosomal acid lipase activity: A new marker of liver disease severity across the clinical continuum of non-alcoholic fatty liver disease? World Journal of Gastroenterology. 2019;**25**(30):4172-4180. DOI: 10.3748/wjg.v25.i30.4172

[63] Carotti S, Aquilano K, Valentini F, et al. An overview of deregulated lipid metabolism in nonalcoholic fatty liver disease with special focus on lysosomal acid lipase. American Journal of Physiology. Gastrointestinal and Liver Physiology. 2020;**319**(4):G469-G480. DOI: 10.1152/ajpgi.00049.2020

[64] Schott MB, Weller SG, Schulze RJ, et al. Lipid droplet size directs lipolysis and lipophagy catabolism in hepatocytes. The Journal of Cell Biology. 2019;**218**(10):3320-3335. DOI: 10.1083/jcb.201803153

[65] Mashek DG. Hepatic lipid droplets: A balancing act between energy storage and metabolic dysfunction in NAFLD. Molecular Metabolism. 2021;**50**:101115. DOI: 10.1016/j.molmet.2020.101115

[66] Qian H, Chao X, Williams J, et al. Autophagy in liver diseases: A review. Molecular Aspects of Medicine. 2021;**82**:100973. DOI: 10.1016/j.mam.2021.100973

[67] Schulze RJ, Krueger EW, Weller SG, et al. Direct lysosome-based autophagy of lipid droplets in hepatocytes. Proceedings of the National Academy of Sciences of the United States of America. 2020;**117**(51):32443-32452. DOI: 10.1073/pnas.2011442117

[68] Sathyanarayan A, Mashek MT, Mashek DG. ATGL promotes autophagy/lipophagy via SIRT1 to control hepatic lipid droplet catabolism. Cell Reports. 2017;**19**(1):1-9. DOI: 10.1016/j.celrep.2017.03.026

[69] Koga H, Kaushik S, Cuervo AM. Altered lipid content inhibits autophagic vesicular fusion. The FASEB Journal.

2010;**24**(8):3052-3065. DOI: 10.1096/fj.09-144519

[70] Challa TD, Wueest S, Lucchini FC, et al. Liver ASK1 protects from non-alcoholic fatty liver disease and fibrosis. EMBO Molecular Medicine. 2019;**11**(10):e10124. DOI: 10.15252/emmm.201810124

[71] Wang Y, Wen H, Fu J, et al. Hepatocyte TNF receptor-associated factor 6 aggravates hepatic inflammation and fibrosis by promoting lysine 6-linked Polyubiquitination of apoptosis signal-regulating kinase 1. Hepatology. 2020;**71**(1):93-111. DOI: 10.1002/hep.30822

[72] Wang CW, Miao YH, Chang YS. A sterol-enriched vacuolar microdomain mediates stationary phase lipophagy in budding yeast. The Journal of Cell Biology. 2014;**206**(3):357-366. DOI: 10.1083/jcb.201404115

[73] Tsuji T, Fujimoto M, Tatematsu T, et al. Niemann-pick type C proteins promote microautophagy by expanding raft-like membrane domains in the yeast vacuole. eLife. 2017;**6**:e25960. DOI: 10.7554/eLife.25960

[74] Oku M, Maeda Y, Kagohashi Y, et al. Evidence for ESCRT- and clathrin-dependent microautophagy. The Journal of Cell Biology. 2017;**216**(10):3263-3274. DOI: 10.1083/jcb.201611029

[75] Szántó M, Gupte R, Kraus WL, et al. PARPs in lipid metabolism and related diseases. Progress in Lipid Research. 2021;**84**:101117. DOI: 10.1016/j.plipres.2021.101117

[76] Ipsen DH, Lykkesfeldt J, Tveden-Nyborg P. Molecular mechanisms of hepatic lipid accumulation in non-alcoholic fatty liver disease. Cellular and Molecular Life Sciences. 2018;**75**(18):3313-3327. DOI: 10.1007/s00018-018-2860-6

[77] Gao Q, Jia Y, Yang G, et al. PPARα-deficient ob/ob obese mice become more obese and manifest severe hepatic steatosis due to decreased fatty acid oxidation. The American Journal of Pathology. 2015;**185**(5):1396-1408. DOI: 10.1016/j.ajpath.2015.01.018

[78] von Loeffelholz C, Döcke S, Lock JF, et al. Increased lipogenesis in spite of upregulated hepatic 5'AMP-activated protein kinase in human non-alcoholic fatty liver. Hepatology Research. 2017;**47**(9):890-901. DOI: 10.1111/hepr.12825

[79] Hodson L, Gunn PJ. The regulation of hepatic fatty acid synthesis and partitioning: The effect of nutritional state. Nature Reviews Endocrinology. 2019;**15**(12):689-700. DOI: 10.1038/s41574-019-0256-9

[80] Moore MP, Cunningham RP, Meers GM, et al. Compromised hepatic mitochondrial fatty acid oxidation and reduced markers of mitochondrial turnover in human NAFLD. Hepatology. 2022. DOI: 10.1002/hep.32324 [Online]

[81] Heeren J, Scheja L. Metabolic-associated fatty liver disease and lipoprotein metabolism. Molecular Metabolism. 2021;**50**:101238. DOI: 10.1016/j.molmet.2021.101238

[82] Alves-Bezerra M, Cohen DE. Triglyceride metabolism in the liver. Comprehensive Physiology. 2017;**8**(1):1-8. DOI: 10.1002/cphy.c170012

[83] Santos-Baez LS, Ginsberg HN. Nonalcohol fatty liver disease: Balancing supply and utilization of triglycerides. Current Opinion in Lipidology.

2021;**32**(3):200-206. DOI: 10.1097/MOL.0000000000000756

[84] Kawano Y, Cohen DE. Mechanisms of hepatic triglyceride accumulation in non-alcoholic fatty liver disease. Journal of Gastroenterology. 2013;**48**(4):434-441. DOI: 10.1007/s00535-013-0758-5

[85] Fabbrini E, Mohammed BS, Magkos F, et al. Alterations in adipose tissue and hepatic lipid kinetics in obese men and women with nonalcoholic fatty liver disease. Gastroenterology. 2008;**134**(2):424-431. DOI: 10.1053/j.gastro.2007.11.038

[86] Umpleby AM, Shojaee-Moradie F, Fielding B, et al. Impact of liver fat on the differential partitioning of hepatic triacylglycerol into VLDL subclasses on high and low sugar diets. Clinical Science (London, England). 2017;**131**(21):2561-2573. DOI: 10.1042/CS20171208

[87] Gill JM, Brown JC, Caslake MJ, et al. Effects of dietary monounsaturated fatty acids on lipoprotein concentrations, compositions, and subfraction distributions and on VLDL apolipoprotein B kinetics: Dose-dependent effects on LDL. The American Journal of Clinical Nutrition. 2003;**78**(1):47-56. DOI: 10.1093/ajcn/78.1.47

[88] Parks EJ, Krauss RM, Christiansen MP, et al. Effects of a low-fat, high-carbohydrate diet on VLDL-triglyceride assembly, production, and clearance. The Journal of Clinical Investigation. 1999;**104**(8):1087-1096. DOI: 10.1172/JCI6572

[89] Yu Y, Cai J, She Z, et al. Insights into the epidemiology, pathogenesis, and therapeutics of nonalcoholic fatty liver diseases. Advanced Science (Weinh). 2018;**6**(4):1801585. DOI: 10.1002/advs.201801585

[90] Loomba R. Role of imaging-based biomarkers in NAFLD: Recent advances in clinical application and future research directions. Journal of Hepatology. 2018;**68**(2):296-304. DOI: 10.1016/j.jhep.2017.11.028

[91] Puri P, Xu J, Vihervaara T, et al. Alcohol produces distinct hepatic lipidome and eicosanoid signature in lean and obese. Journal of Lipid Research. 2016;**57**(6):1017-1028. DOI: 10.1194/jlr.M066175

[92] Wang M, Palavicini JP, Cseresznye A, et al. Strategy for quantitative analysis of isomeric Bis(monoacylglycero) phosphate and Phosphatidylglycerol species by shotgun Lipidomics after one-step methylation. Analytical Chemistry. 2017;**89**(16):8490-8495. DOI: 10.1021/acs.analchem.7b02058

[93] Ščupáková K, Soons Z, Ertaylan G, et al. Spatial systems Lipidomics reveals nonalcoholic fatty liver disease heterogeneity. Analytical Chemistry. 2018;**90**(8):5130-5138. DOI: 10.1021/acs.analchem.7b05215

[94] Patterson RE, Kirpich AS, Koelmel JP, et al. Improved experimental data processing for UHPLC–HRMS/MS lipidomics applied to nonalcoholic fatty liver disease. Metabolomics. 2017;**142**. DOI: 10.1007/s11306-017-1280-1

[95] Hatori M, Vollmers C, Zarrinpar A, et al. Time-restricted feeding without reducing caloric intake prevents metabolic diseases in mice fed a high-fat diet. Cell Metabolism. 2012;**15**(6):848-860. DOI: 10.1016/j.cmet.2012.04.019

[96] Baumeier C, Kaiser D, Heeren J, et al. Caloric restriction and intermittent fasting alter hepatic lipid droplet proteome and diacylglycerol species and prevent diabetes in NZO mice. Biochimica et Biophysica Acta.

2015;**1851**(5):566-576. DOI: 10.1016/j.bbalip.2015.01.013

[97] Musso G, Cassader M, Rosina F, et al. Impact of current treatments on liver disease, glucose metabolism and cardiovascular risk in non-alcoholic fatty liver disease (NAFLD): A systematic review and meta-analysis of randomised trials. Diabetologia. 2012;**55**(4):885-904. DOI: 10.1007/s00125-011-2446-4

[98] Li C, Li L, Lian J, et al. Roles of acyl-CoA: Diacylglycerol acyltransferases 1 and 2 in triacylglycerol synthesis and secretion in primary hepatocytes. Arteriosclerosis, Thrombosis, and Vascular Biology. 2015;**35**(5):1080-1091. DOI: 10.1161/ATVBAHA.114.304584

[99] Stiede K, Miao W, Blanchette HS, et al. Acetyl-coenzyme A carboxylase inhibition reduces de novo lipogenesis in overweight male subjects: A randomized, double-blind, crossover study. Hepatology. 2017;**66**(2):324-334. DOI: 10.1002/hep.29246

[100] Reddy JK, Rao MS. Lipid metabolism and liver inflammation. II. Fatty liver disease and fatty acid oxidation. American Journal of Physiology. Gastrointestinal and Liver Physiology. 2006;**290**(5):G852-G858. DOI: 10.1152/ajpgi.00521.2005

[101] Hazlehurst JM, Woods C, Marjot T, et al. Non-alcoholic fatty liver disease and diabetes. Metabolism. 2016;**65**(8):1096-1108. DOI: 10.1016/j.metabol.2016.01.001

[102] Jain MR, Giri SR, Trivedi C, et al. Saroglitazar, a novel PPARα/γ agonist with predominant PPARα activity, shows lipid-lowering and insulin-sensitizing effects in preclinical models. Pharmacology Research & Perspectives. 2015;**3**(3):e00136. DOI: 10.1002/prp2.136

[103] Musa-Veloso K, Venditti C, Lee HY, et al. Systematic review and meta-analysis of controlled intervention studies on the effectiveness of long-chain omega-3 fatty acids in patients with nonalcoholic fatty liver disease. Nutrition Reviews. 2018;**76**(8):581-602. DOI: 10.1093/nutrit/nuy022

Chapter 3

Transcriptional Regulation by ERR and Its Role in NAFLD Pathogenesis

Brittney Hua, Ielyzaveta Slarve, Aditi A. Datta, Chenxi Xu, Chien-yu Chen and Bangyan L. Stiles

Abstract

Members of estrogen-related receptors (ERRs) are orphan nuclear receptors (NRs) that play primary roles in mitochondrial biogenesis and bioenergetics. The ERRs regulate a range of cellular functions, including oxidative phosphorylation (OXPHOS) as well as glucose and lipid metabolism. ERRs are considered important targets for the treatment of metabolic diseases, particularly type II diabetes (T2D), insulin resistance (IR) and obesity. In this review, we will overview the transcriptional network regulated by the members of ERR transcriptional factors and elaborate on the regulation of ERR via its binding to PGC-1α, the primary co-activator of ERR as well as post-translational regulation of ERRs by upstream kinase signals. Recent development in ERR's cellular function has identified lipid metabolism/lipogenesis as a process that ERR regulates, and this function significantly impacts metabolic syndrome. Here, we will focus on their roles in lipid metabolic regulation and discuss the *in vivo* functions of ERRs in the development of non-alcoholic fatty liver disease (NAFLD), a comorbid metabolic syndrome concurrent with T2D, IR as well as obesity. Finally, we will explore ERRs as potential therapeutic targets by discussing the ligands that serve as antagonist/agonists for ERRs as well as efforts that target DNA binding of ERR as a transcriptional factor.

Keywords: estrogen receptor, nuclear receptor, energy metabolism, metabolic syndrome, mitochondria, fatty liver

1. Introduction

The ERR family of transcription factors are orphan NRs that are characterized for their functions in the transcriptional regulation of genes involved in mitochondrial bioenergetics and function [1]. Members of the ERR family orphan NRs regulate a range of cellular functions, including OXPHOS as well as glucose and lipid metabolism [2] and play critical roles in the transcriptional regulation of genes involved in mitochondrial bioenergetics, TCA cycle, mitochondrial OXPHOS, and fatty acid β-oxidation [3]. The ERRs in general serve as positive transcriptional regulators of genes regulating mitochondrial respiration and negative regulators for genes regulating gluconeogenesis [4–6]. These properties make ERRs potential targets for understanding and treating metabolic diseases, particularly T2D, IR, and obesity. In this review, we will summarize the overall function of ERRs and their regulations. We will then focus on their roles in the development of liver steatosis, particularly NAFLD and non-alcoholic steatohepatitis (NASH).

2. Discovery of ERRs

ERR was first identified during the efforts of searching for isoforms of estrogen receptors (ER) using a reduced stringency hybridization protocol to screen recombinant DNA libraries and discover novel receptors [7]. In this screening, the estrogen receptor DNA-binding domain (DBD) was used as the hybridization probe to screen the human testis cDNA library. This screening resulted in the identification of three positive clones of which two encoded for known ERs. The third clone demonstrated partial sequence similarity with ER. This sequence was later identified as a novel receptor and termed the ERRs [7]. Like other NRs, members of the ERR family contain six conserved functional domain structures (A-F) [8, 9]. The most highly conserved region is the C domain, which contains the DBD. This domain is composed of two highly conserved zinc finger motifs, CI and CII, which are DNA-binding motifs that allow ERR to bind to the estrogen related response element (ERRE), which contains the hexanucleotide DNA sequence 5′AGGTCA-3′ that is also recognized by ER [10] (**Figure 1**). The ERRs are able to bind to ERRE as either monomers, homodimers, or heterodimers. The A/B domain located at the N-terminal, is also referred to as the activation-function-1 (AF-1) domain that is ligand-independent. This domain is the least conserved region compared to other NRs, and its activation capacity varies between different NRs [11]. The D domain contains the hinge region that is needed for receptor dimerization and is also involved in the interaction of ERR

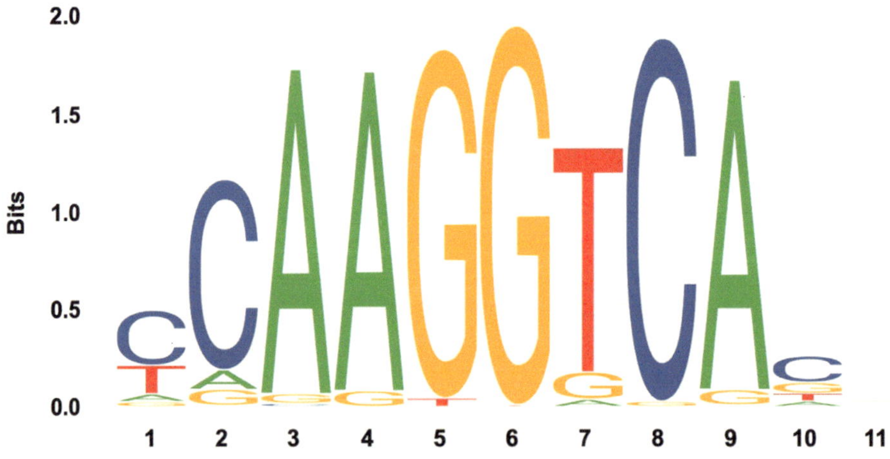

Figure 1.
ERRE binding motif sequence for ERR. JASPAR2022 database was used to generate a logo of the DNA binding motif sequence for ERR. The total height of the letters C, G, T and A at each position was derived from the mean information content available from a collection of transcription factor binding sites in units of bits (y-axis). The height of each letter is representative of the nucleotide frequency in a specific position (x-axis) in the aligned promoter sequence. The three isoforms of human estrogen related receptors have the consensus DNA sequence 5′AGGTCA-3′, which is referred to as the estrogen related receptor response element (ERRE).

with co-regulatory proteins [12]. The E/F domain located at the C-terminal contains the ligand binding domain (LBD). Once a ligand binds to the receptor, ligand-induced conformational changes to the LBD occur, and the ligand becomes trapped in the hydrophobic-binding pocket from the hydrophobic core of the LBD [12–14]. The LBD is also part of the AF-2 domain that is ligand-dependent. The full transcriptional activity for a NR requires the synergistic cooperation between AF-1 and AF-2 [11].

The DBD of ERR shares 54–68% amino acid homology with other known NRs including ER, but with very little target gene similarities [8, 15]. While structurally similar to ER, ERRs preferentially bind to 5′-TCAAGGTCA-3′ rather than the direct repeat sequence of two hexanucleotide sequence of 5′-AGGTCA-3′ that is preferentially recognized by ER [10]. This ERRE sequence represents a 3 bp 5′ extension of the classical hexanucleotide repeat response elements for classical nuclear receptors. Such response elements have been observed for receptors that bind to DNA as monomers, including the rev-Erb and retinoid-related orphan receptors among others. Thus, ERR is expected to be capable of binding to ERRE as a monomer. In addition, ERRs also share high LBD sequence similarity with ERs. However, despite the high sequence and structure similarities of the LBD, studies have found that ERR is unable to bind to estrogen as endogenous ligands. Crystal structures of the coactivator bound LBD domains of ERR show that they adopt an active conformation without the binding of a ligand [16–18]. This conformation is similar in structure as the estrogen bound active ERα. The putative ligand binding pocket formed by the LBD domains of ERR appears to be the smallest observed among nuclear receptors and can only accommodate a structure that is half the size of estrogen. In addition, docking studies show that steric hindrance of D ring on estrogen with L345 and F435, precludes binding of estrogen to ERR in the active conformation.

3. Estrogen related receptor (ERR) family of transcriptional factors and the transcriptional networks they regulate

3.1 Regulation of estrogen-responsive genes by ERRs

Despite their sequence homology (36%) with ERs in the LBD, ERRs do not (or only very weakly) respond to estradiol (E2) and are constitutively active [18–22]. Their LBD interacts with the steroid receptor coactivator 1 (SRC-1) in the absence of any ligand and resumes an active conformation [18]. Since ERRs are identified using DBD of ER and the two receptors share high DBD domain similarities, all three members of the ERR family are able to bind to the half-site hexanucleotide repeat of the classical estrogen response element (ERE) that are recognized by ER [8]. Because of these characteristics of ERRs, earlier studies focused on identifying target genes that are shared by ERR and ER. These studies identified a small handful of genes of which the transcriptions are co-regulated by ERR and ER [23–25]. These genes were associated with clinical outcomes in a COX regression analysis. Among them, pS2, a well-recognized marker for breast cancer was the first common ERR and ER target identified [25]. It was demonstrated that ERRα is a transcriptional activator that interacts with coactivators and binds to EREs in the absence of a ligand in ER+ breast cancers. This ERR induced activity was accredited for the ability of diethylstilbestrol, an ER/ERR antagonist to inhibit pS2 expression in ER- breast cancer cells. Using luciferase reporters in ER+ MCF-7 cells, it was shown that the ERRα competes with ER for binding to ERE and acts as a repressor for the transcription regulation of ER responsive genes. On the other hand, ERRα acts as a transcription activator in Hela cells when ER and estrogen are not present [13].

3.2 Isoform specific transcriptional regulation by members of the ERR family of transcriptional factors

The ERR subfamily of nuclear receptors comprises three members: ERRα (NR3B1), ERRβ (NR3B2), and ERRγ (NR3B3), with all members having high amino acid sequence homology. ERRβ and ERRγ have high conservations in their LBD domain, where they share less similarities with ERRα. A distinct difference in ERRα is the presence of a phenylalanine at F382 that significantly alters the size and shape of the ligand binding pocket. As a result, ERRα cannot bind to 4-hydroxytamoxifen which acts as antagonist for ERRβ, γ as well as ERs. ERRα, the first orphan nuclear receptor identified from its close homology to Erα [26], is ubiquitously expressed in all cells and tissues, and highly expressed in high oxidative organs. In these tissues/cells, ERRα regulates the expression of genes involved in glycolysis, such as glyceraldehyde dehydrogenase (GAPDH), and binds to the glucose transporter family members [27]. In breast cancer cells, decreased uptake of glucose is observed in the absence of ERRα [28]. Therefore, ERRα is recognized as an important transcriptional activator for cellular glucose metabolism in response to environmental stimuli [29].

In addition, ERRα is identified as the key transcriptional factor for the regulation of OXPHOS [19–22]. Using mouse myocytes to screen for cis-regulatory elements responsible for the regulation of OXPHOS by PCG-1α and β (Peroxisomal proliferation activated receptor γ (PPARγ) coactivator-1), ERRα was identified together with a ETS family of transcription regulators. In this study, 20 common motifs are identified from over 5000 differentially expressed genes induced by the exogenous expression of PGC-1α (1–3 days) [20]. A majority of the 20 motifs, particularly those that displayed changes early in days 1 and 2, are related to ERR regulated promoters. The ERR motifs are found in >50% of the OXPHOS genes coregulated by PGC-1α. Supporting this analysis, a study performed in livers from type 2 diabetes patients identified ERRα and PPARγ as the two nuclear factors correlated with OXPHOS and can be used as predictors for fasting glucose levels [19]. Adenovirus-mediated expression of PGC-1α in ERRα positive and negative mouse embryonic fibroblasts (mEFs) derived showed that genes regulating mitochondrial functions were among the primary transcripts differentially regulated when ERRα is lost [30]. In particular, the inability of PGC-1α to induce citrate synthase activity, a key indicator of mitochondrial activity in the absence of ERRα supports the role of ERRα in the regulation of mitochondrial function.

ERRα regulates the expression of genes that form the mitochondrial respiratory system, including those that encode proteins involved in the TCA mitochondrial oxidative phosphorylation, respiratory chain, and TCA cycle (**Figure 2**). In addition to regulating the expression of genes encoding mitochondrial proteins, inhibition of ERRα also diminishes the ability of PGC-1α to increase mitochondrial DNA content [21]. In SAOS2 cells where PGC-1α induces mitochondrial biogenesis and function, ERRα is needed for sustaining the expression of TFAM, a mitochondrial transcriptional factor that induces mitochondrial DNA replication and transcription, Tim22, a core translocase protein responsible for the integrity of mitochondrial inner membrane proteins, isocitrate dehydrogenase α, which catalyzes the irreversible oxidative decarboxylation of isocitrate to yield α-ketoglutarate (α-KG) and CO2 as part of the TCA cycle, carnitine/acylcarnitine translocase, the rate limiting enzyme for fatty

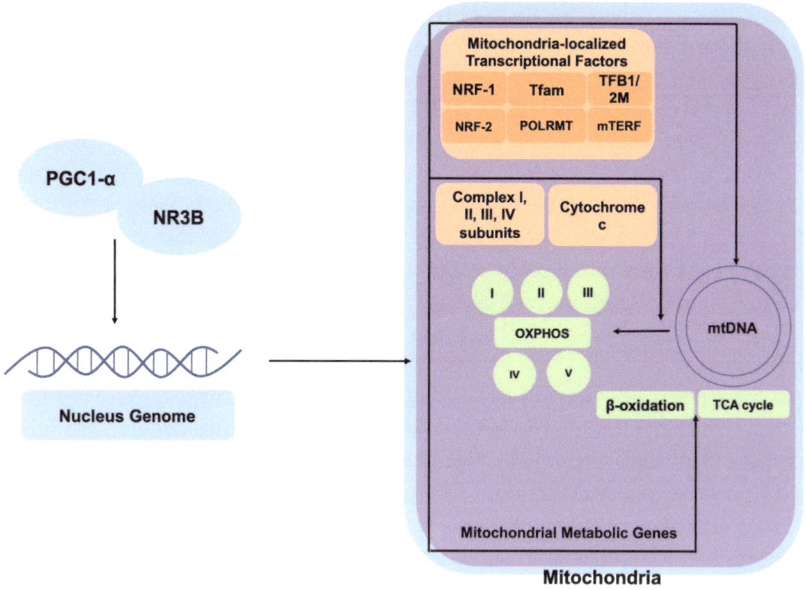

Figure 2.
ERR is a master regulator for mitochondrial functions and biogenesis. ERR regulates the gene expression of metabolic enzymes and mitochondrial respiratory complexes in the nucleus and mitochondria. PGC-1α binds to NR3B as a coactivator, entering subsequent transcriptional process. It further impacts transcriptional factors such as NRF-1/2, TFAM, POLRMT, TFB1/2M, METERF. Mitochondrial DNA (mtDNA) transcriptional activity is then activated. Meanwhile, genes encode proteins involved in mitochondrial oxidative phosphorylation, respiratory chain, and TCA cycle, including cytochrome C (Cytc), NADH dehydrogenase are regulated as well.

acid oxidation, as well as Cytochrome *c* and ATP synβ, both directly involved in the electron transportation during OXPHOS [21].

The role of ERRα as a regulator of mitochondrial function and OXPHOS is validated in neonatal cardiomyocytes, where a significant number of genes induced by ERRα expression are involved in cellular energy metabolic pathways [22]. In addition, a number of genes involved in mitochondrial fatty acid oxidation and lipid uptake are also induced by ERRα overexpression. Notably, medium chain acyl-CoA decarboxylase (MCAD), the rate limiting enzyme involved in fatty acid β-oxidation was confirmed as a direct transcriptional target for ERR by several other studies as well [10, 22].

Despite the differences in LBD, gene-chip analysis shows that ERRα and ERRγ target a common set of promoters of genes related to OXPHOS and fatty acid oxidation [31, 32]. In this context, both ERRs serve as positive transcriptional regulators of genes regulating mitochondrial respiration and fatty acid oxidation as well regulators for genes involved in gluconeogenesis [31, 33, 34]. In addition, ERRγ also positively regulate the promoters of G6Pasc and PEPCK, two rate limiting enzymes of gluconeogenesis, while ERRα has been shown to be the transcriptional repressor of PEPCK [34]. ERRγ, the newest member identified in the ERR superfamily, plays a role in controlling metabolic switching in the perinatal heart and acts as a direct transcriptional regulator of GATA4 [35]. Compared to ERRα, which is associated with poor breast cancer outcomes, the overexpression of ERRγ was reported to associate with a better prognosis [36]. ERRγ was also identified as a potential tumor suppressor in gastric cancer by negatively regulating the Wnt signaling pathway [37]. Similar to ERRα, ERRγ plays a role in the regulation of mitochondrial gene expression [38].

In recent years, a role of ERRs in pluripotency has been identified primarily through studies of reprogramming of somatic cells to immortalized pluripotent stem cells (iPS) [39–41]. This was first recognized with ERRβ, which was found to replace Nanog or Klf4 during reprograming of iPS [39, 42]. In particular, ERRβ was found to bind to many target sites co-occupied by OCT4-SOX2-Nanog (OSN) [40, 41, 43], the transcriptional network characterized for their functions in maintaining "stemness". ERRβ participates in the regulation of these factors and their targets and is also a direct transcriptional target of Nanog [39]. Conversely, ERRβ also interacts with Oct4 within the *Nanog* promoter, a component also regulated by the Wnt/Gsk3 pathway [27, 41]. Further studies show that ERRβ is regulated by leukemia inhibitory factor (LIF), Wnt, PROX1, Ncoa3 as well as nucleostemin [44–48], all involved in pluripotency regulation.

In vivo, ERRβ is highly expressed during embryogenesis and is involved in the development and physiologic function of different tissues and organs, including the placenta, inner ear, and retina [49]. Embryos carrying homozygous deletions of ERRβ displayed impaired placental formation and died *in utero*, indicating that ERRβ plays a crucial role during early placental stages [50]. Consistently, knockdown or knockout of ERR allows for differentiation and calcium deposition while suppressing expression of genes associates with progenitor cells [51–53].

It was later reported that all three ERR isoforms are capable of supporting iPS reprogramming [54]. Using ERRα and γ and their cofactors to induce OXPHOS, it was demonstrated that at least an initial burst of the OXPHOS activity is necessary for the reprogramming of iPS [54]. ERRβ also regulates OXPHOS, similar to ERRα and γ [55]. Together, this work established that ERR transcriptional factors and the transcriptional network regulated by ERRs play an important role in the regulation of cell fate.

4. Regulation of ERRα

4.1 Regulation via binding with co-activator PGC-1

Like other NRs, ERRs bind to co-activators for their functions. Although the p160 family of coactivator SRC-1 was used to co-crystalize with LBD of ERRγ, the p160 family of coactivators only weakly bind with ERRs. On the other hand, ERRα is identified as one of the primary partner for PGC-1α in the regulation of mitochondrial biogenesis [56]. PGC-1 was discovered to bind both ERRα and γ via a LXXLL motif that is also necessary for PGC-1 to bind other nuclear receptors [57]. The AF-2 domains on ERRs are needed for this binding to occur. PGC-1 is highly expressed in tissues with high energy demands including heart, kidney, brown fat, and muscle [58], similar to the tissue distribution of ERRα and γ. Studies suggest that PGC-1 can be considered as the protein "ligand" for ERR since there is no endogenous lipophilic ligand identified for ERRs [59]. Binding to PGC-1α turns ERRα from a weak to a strong transcriptional factor. This is achieved by directly increasing of ERRα expression as PGC-1α-ERRα complex binds to the promoters of ERRα itself [60, 61]. In addition, cofactor binding allows ERRs to assume active conformation and increase its activity as a transcriptional factor [16, 62]. Together, the PGC-1α-ERR complex activates genes that encode proteins critical for mitochondrial components or activating transcription factors involved in mitochondrial biogenesis. In addition, PGC-1β, another isoform of PGC-1 coactivators that is often considered regulators of basal mitochondrial biogenesis, has also been reported to bind and regulate the transcriptional activities of ERRs.

PGCs are originally identified as transcriptional coactivators of PPARγ for adaptive thermogenesis in response to cold induction [58]. All three members of the PGC family (PGC-1α, PGC-1β and PRC) of coactivators play roles in mitochondrial biogenesis by regulating the expression of overlapping genes. Unlike the p160 family of coactivators, PGC-1 family of coactivators does not possess histone acetyltransferase activities. Instead, they provide docking sites for histone acetyltransferases including SRC-1 as well as CBP/p300 [63]. PGC-1α responds to different stimuli to induce mitochondrial biogenesis via binding to ERRs as well as others nuclear receptors such as PPARγ and nuclear respiratory factors (NRF). PGC-1 s also have the capacity to bind other transcriptional factor including the forkhead and the yin-yang transcriptional factors among others [6]. Thus, the activity of these transcription factors including ERRs are coordinately coregulated through their competition and coordination in binding to PGC-1. In addition, the binding of PGC-1α to ERRs and other nuclear factors is regulated by Prox1, a homeobox protein that is tethered with ERRs and other nuclear factors to participate in their transcriptional activity [44].

PGC-1 s are subject themselves to post-translational regulation, and these regulations play important roles in their response to different stimuli. In general, PGC-1α responds to the different stimuli and is regulated by cell signaling pathways to control mitochondrial biogenesis and function. Notably, AMP activated kinase (AMPK) phosphorylates PGC-1α on Thr177 and Ser 538 and increases its transcriptional activity [64]. On the other hand, PGC-1α phosphorylation by AKT or S6K integrates nutrient signals to suppress its gluconeogenesis and activity towards fatty acid oxidation [65, 66]. PGC-1α also cross-talks with the sirtuin family of protein deacetylases to regulate metabolism. PGC-1α is activated by SIRT1-mediated deacetylation when cells sense changes of NAD+/NADH ratios [67]. In addition, PGC-1α is also methylated and ubiquitinated to meet different cellular energy demands [68].

4.2 Post-translational modifications and signaling

In MCF-7 cells, treatment of epidermal growth factor (EGF) leads to phosphorylation of ERRα and enhances its transcriptional activity [69]. In this study, PKCd was found capable of phosphorylating ERRα on the DBD, resulting in its enrichment at the ERRE containing promoters [69]. Screening breast cancer samples for expression of ER and ERR isoforms identified ERRα as the potential biomarker for poor prognosis for ER- and ErbB2 high expressing tumors [36]. In MCF-7 cells, overexpression of ErbB2 leads to hyperphosphorylation of ERRα and increased transcriptional activity [70]. This ErbB2 induced phosphorylation is readily inhibited by anti-ErbB2 as well as U0126 and LY294002, inhibitors for MAP kinase and AKT, two major signaling kinases downstream of ErbB2 signaling pathway. *In vitro*, both MAPK and AKT were found to phosphorylate AKT. Multiple phospho-sites are found throughout the protein for MAPK and phospho-sites for AKT are also predicted based on these in vitro kinase studies. However, no phospho-site has been identified thus far for each of the kinases.

Being the downstream signal induced by insulin signal, the PI3K/AKT signal plays major roles in regulating glucose metabolism, including glycolysis, gluconeogenesis as well as the TCA cycle and mitochondrial functions [71] (**Figure 3**). In hepatocytes and livers where PI3K/AKT signal is induced due to loss of negative regulator phosphatase and tensin homolog deleted on chromosome 10 (PTEN) expression, upregulation of ERRα as well as OXPHOS are observed [72]. Activation of PI3K/AKT leads to increased oxygen consumption (OCR) as well as induction of mitochondrial biogenesis [72, 73], whereas inhibiting ERRα activity blocks the induction of

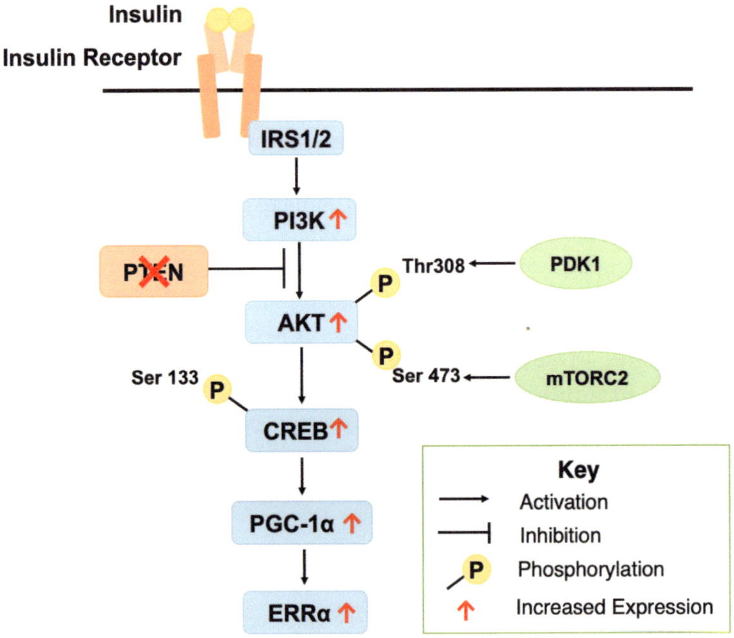

Figure 3.
PI3K/AKT signalling regulates ERRα. Activation and phosphorylation of insulin receptors results in recruitment of PI3K and the subsequent conversion of phosphatidylinositol (3,4)-biphosphate (PIP_2) to phosphatidylinositol (3,4,5)-triphosphate (PIP_3). PTEN, a negative regulator of the PI3K/AKT pathway, converts PIP_3 back to PIP_2. Following binding to PIP_3, the serine/threonine kinase AKT becomes fully activated via phosphorylation at Thr308 and Ser473 by 3-phosphoinositide-dependent kinase 1 (PDK1) and mammalian target of rapamycin complex 2 (mTORC2), respectively. Activated AKT then phosphorylates various downstream substrates, including forkhead box O (FOXO) transcription factors, glycogen synthase kinase-3 (GSK3α/β), and tuberous sclerosis complex-2 (TSC2), a critical negative regulator of mTORC1 signaling. Activated AKT also phosphorylates CREB at Ser133, leading to an increase in PGC-1α and ERRα expression.

mitochondrial function by PI3K/AKT signal [72]. Phosphorylation of CREB by AKT is thought to play a role in the regulation of ERRα by AKT in these cells, though direct phosphorylation of ERRα by AKT cannot be ruled out.

Due to the lack of endogenous ligands identified, ERRα is thought to be regulated primarily via transactivation and by upstream signaling pathways. However, not much has been elucidated for post-translation modification of ERRs beyond the reported phosphorylation of ERRα associated with breast cancer cell growth and survival. One addition modification reported is sumoylation at lysine 14 (Lys14), which suppresses its transcriptional activity with unexplored mechanisms [74]. It was found that this sumoylation of ERRα is dependent on its phosphorylation at serine 19 (Ser19).

The discovery of the roles ERR play in iPS have led to studies exploring how ERR signals crosstalk with those regulating pluripotency. These studies led to the discovery that ERRα physically interacts with β-catenin and lymphoid enhanced-binding factor-1 (LEF-1), with an overlap among genes previously demonstrated to be regulated by either β-catenin or ERRα [75]. A reduction of migratory capacity of breast, prostate, and colon cancer cell lines was observed following silencing of either β-catenin or ERRα with siRNAs, and this effect was further enhanced when the expression of both proteins was reduced simultaneously. The increased migratory capacity of cancer cells was suggested to occur as a result of the ERRα/β-catenin-dependent induction of Wnt 11, an activator of noncanonical Wnt signaling pathway [75]. Furthermore, ERRα is also reported to regulate osteoblast differentiation via the Wnt/β-catenin signaling pathway. In C3H10T1/2 cells overexpression of ERRα with PGC-1α or overexpression of Wnt3a, a significant overlap in gene expression is observed. These results suggest that the expression of ERRα and PGC-1α causes similar gene changes within the Wnt pathway as activation by Wnt3a alone [51].

5. The role of ERR in lipid metabolism

The functions of ERRs have been defined by their interactions with PGC-1 s as coactivators. Beside inducing OXPHOS and supply the cellular energy demand, ERRs also activate transcription of numerous genes involved in oxidative metabolism that depends on mitochondrial respiration. ERRE is located in the promoter region of the gene that encodes carnitine-acylcarnitine carrier (SLC25A29), which is involved in the net transport of fatty acyl units to the mitochondrial matrix, where they are oxidized through β-oxidation. In addition, ERRE is located in the 5′-flanking region of the gene encoding for MCAD, a key enzyme involved in the initial step of mitochondrial β-oxidation [10]. AMPK-mediated expression of ERRα and PGC-1β and subsequent expression of MCAD/CPT1 is found to play a role in fatty acid β-oxidation in tamoxifen-resistant MCF-7 cells.

Genetic deletion of ERRα or ERRγ in mice confirmed the role of these ERRs in mitochondrial biogenesis and oxidative capacity, particularly in tissues with high energy demand [26, 76]. In cardiac muscles and brown adipose tissue where mitochondrial biogenesis and bioenergetic is needed for the function of the tissue, impaired adaptation to hemodynamic stressors and thermogenesis is observed respectively when ERRα is lost [77, 78]. Loss of ERRγ also resulted in the failure to switch to a oxidative transcriptome [76].

Given these positive regulatory roles of ERRs in mitochondrial respiration and fatty acid oxidation, loss of ERRs is expected to inhibit catabolic metabolism. However, deletion of ERRα, while viable and fertile, exhibited reduced fat mass and resistant to high-fat diet induced obesity [26]. Although mice lacking ERRβ or ERRγ are not viable to adulthood due to placenta and cardiac failures respectively [50, 58, 61, 76], pharmacological inhibition of either ERRγ (the dominant form of ERR in cardiac and skeletal muscles) or ERRα have led to improved insulin response and better tolerance to diet induced metabolic changes [79, 80]. Consistent with the reduced fat mass phenotype, lipogenic genes such as fatty acid synthase (Fasn) and elongase (Elov3) in the adipose tissue are all inhibited when ERRα is absent [26]. In agreement with this putative function of ERRs in lipogenesis, ERRα and PGC1-α expression are concurrently upregulated in response to adipogenic inductions [81]. ERR and PGC1-α together are found to be required for adipogenic differentiation induced by glucocorticoid, cAMP and insulin [81, 82]. Consistent with these observations, ChIP-on-Chip and ChIP-seq analysis indeed show that ERRα can occupy the promoter regions of Fasn and acetyl-CoA carboxylase (ACC), the two rate-limiting enzymes in the lipogenic pathways [83]. Inhibition of ERRα led to reduced triglyceride (TG) content in the liver accompanied by attenuated expression of Fasn and ACC [84].

The storage of lipid into TG starts with esterification of long-chain fatty acids to glycerol 3-phosphate [85] (**Figure 4**). This committed step is catalyzed by GPATs, the rate-limiting enzymes for the process. Acylation at carbon 1 leads to formation of lysophosphatidic acid (LPA) which is converted to phosphatidic acid (PA) via the action of AGPAT. During biosynthesis of triglycerides, PA is converted to

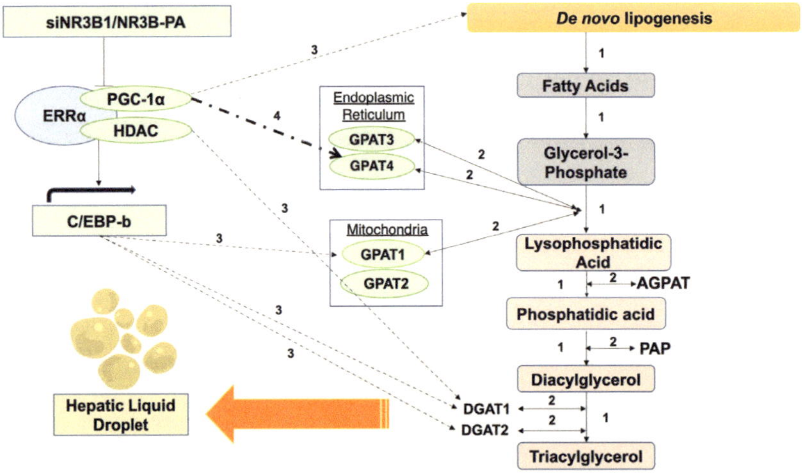

Figure 4.
Glycerolipid biosynthesis pathway. Arrows labeled 1 describe the steps leading to the formation of triacylglycerol. Hepatic de novo lipogenesis results in the synthesis of fatty acids through acylation, which is catalysed by GPAT. G3P and acyl-CoA is converted to lysophosphatidic acid with the help of GPAT. Following this, LPA is converted to phosphatidic acid, which is catalysed by AGPAT. Dephosphorylation of PA by PAP generates diacylglycerol, which further serves as the substrate for DGATs in the synthesis of triglycerides. Arrows labeled 2 indicate a catalysis reaction. Arrows labeled 3 indicate the transcriptional regulation of GPAT enzymes by PGC-1α, and arrow 4 indicates how GPAT4 is transcriptionally regulated by ERRα and co-activator PGC-1α.

diacylglyceride (DAG) via the actions of LIPIN, a group of enzymes recently gained significant attention relating to their functions in lipid particle formation and autophagy. The final step of TG biosynthesis is catalyzed by the actions of DGATs. The preferentially ERRE binding motif, which has a high frequency of 5′GGTCA-3′ was screened for and found in the promoters of *Esrra*, *Dgat1*, *Gpat4*, *Agpat1* and *Agpat3*. Histone marks were also recognized for *Esrra*, *Dgat1*, and *Gpat4*, suggesting that ERRα is being recruited near the transcription initiation sites [84].

Together, these studies thus suggest that ERRα is a broad spectrum of regulator for lipid metabolism including fatty acid b-oxidation, *de novo* lipogenesis as well as glycerolipid biosynthesis. However, how ERRα may play roles in lipid metabolism may be dependent on the metabolic state and physiological stimuli. For example, in liver steatosis induced by rapamycin treatment, lack of ERRα was shown to impair fatty acid oxidation while buildup of citrate due to downregulation of the TCA cycle is redirected towards lipid biosynthesis [83]. Thus, unexplored transcriptional roles of ERRs, at least ERRα in lipid biosynthesis vs. β-oxidation likely play a role in the *in vivo* phenotype observed with ERR function under different metabolic conditions.

6. ERRs in the development and progression of non-alcoholic steatohepatitis

NAFLD and NASH are common chronic liver conditions and comorbid diseases for more severe liver disease [86, 87]. Simple fatty liver or steatosis is readily reversible while NASH can progress to more morbid forms of liver pathologies. In subsets of patients, the disease can progress to fibrosis/cirrhosis and liver cancer.

Lipid metabolic dysfunctions in the liver is a key contributing factor to the development of liver steatosis [88, 89]. Depending on the metabolic state, different cellular processes contribute to liver steatosis. High fat diet (HFD) induces hyperinsulinemia and hyperglycemia concurrent with glucose intolerance and IR together with NAFLD. During HFD feeding, dietary lipids may directly contribute to steatosis in addition to stimulating *de novo* lipogenesis in the liver. High carbohydrate diet (HCD) feeding, on the other hand, induces liver steatosis via carbohydrate-induced *de novo* lipogenesis. In both diets that induce steatosis, ERRα, the dominant liver isoform of ERRs, is upregulated in the liver [84]. Interestingly, ERRα is also induced in the steatotic livers of EtOH diet fed mice, further indicating a potential role of ERRα in liver steatosis.

In addition to diet induction, steatosis develops in patients with metabolic syndromes, including obesity, IR and Diabetes [86, 87]. As high as 80% of T2D patients exhibit NAFLD/NASH in the liver [87, 90]. Under these pathological conditions, abnormal insulin signals also contribute to liver lipid buildup in addition to the excess lipid and carbohydrate content coming from the diet. In obese individuals and particularly individuals with IR, "selective hepatic insulin resistance" is observed [91], where hyperinsulinemia cannot suppress hepatic gluconeogenesis (resistance) but continues to induce lipogenesis (non-resistance), leading to steatosis in the liver. Previous studies have established that insulin regulates *de novo* lipogenesis by activating phosphoinositide 3-kinases (PI3Ks), lipid kinases involved in the PI3K/AKT/mammalian target of rapamycin (mTOR) signaling [92]. In the livers, loss of PTEN expression, a negative regulator of PI3K/AKT, leads to *de novo* lipogenesis and NAFLD development [93, 94]. Loss of AKT2 resulted in attenuation of lipid and blocked NAFLD development [95–97].

Evidence suggests that the PI3K/AKT signal induces CREB cyclic AMP (cAMP)-response element-binding protein) to activate ERRα and mitochondrial biogenesis and bioenergetics in the hepatocytes [72, 98]. AKT was found to directly phosphorylate CREB at Ser133 as CREB contains a RXX(S/T) sequence that is a potential AKT substrate motif72. CREB is a 43 kDa basic/leucine zipper transcription factor expressed in most tissues. It is suggested to control the expression of over 4000 genes [99], including genes involved in regulation of hepatic glucose and lipid metabolism [100, 101]. Here, PGC-1 was found to be necessary for CREB to induce the gluconeogenesis program [101]. Notably, mice deficient in CREB function are prevented from hepatic lipid accumulation in models of metabolic syndromes such as the Zucker Rat, ob/ob mice, STZ induced T2D, as well as HFD-induced NAFLD [102]. However, loss of CREB function also led to fatty liver development in unchallenged mice [100]. The divergent response of CREB-ERRα regulation in hepatocytes where PI3K/AKT is active vs. inactive may be responsible for this paradoxical observation with CREB deficiency [72]. Consistent with this idea, mice deficient for ERRα (*Esrra−/−* mice) have been reported to be resistant to HFD-induced obesity and steatosis in the liver even though ERRα promotes a catabolic metabolic program [26].

It has been suggested that in addition to promoting TG breakdown during refeeding, ERRα also promotes TG buildup during chronic conditions [84, 103]. In NAFLD induced by rapamycin treatment, however, lack of ERRα was shown to impair fatty acid oxidation, while buildup of citrate due to downregulation of the TCA cycle is redirected towards lipid biosynthesis [83]. Thus, unexplored transcriptional roles of ERRs, at least ERRα in lipid biosynthesis vs. β-oxidation, likely play a role in the *in vivo* phenotype observed with ERR function under these different metabolic conditions. Indeed, in addition to the well characterized target MCAD, lipogenic genes are among the list of lipid metabolic genes that ERR regulates in data collected from a ChIP study, suggesting potential function of ERRs in lipid biosynthesis [44].

7. Therapeutic potential for targeting ERRα in NAFLD treatment

Fatty liver and associated diseases including ASH/NASH are comorbid diseases with diabetes, particularly type 2 diabetes (T2D) which accounts for 95% of all diabetes cases [104]. Fatty liver disease occurs in 80% of T2D patients [87, 90]. While simple fatty liver is readily reversible, NASH can progress to more morbid forms of liver pathologies including fibrosis/cirrhosis and even liver cancer. Currently, there is no therapy besides caloric restriction for the treatment of fatty liver disease [105]. A potential therapy is under development in clinical trials that activates FXR, a bile acid receptor. In a completed clinical trial (NCT01265498), FXR ligand obeticholic acid treatment led to NAFLD resolution in 21% of the subjects vs. 13% in placebo treated subjects after 72 weeks of treatment. While these clinical trials are underway, studies exploring molecules that play roles in liver lipid dysfunction have the potential to discover novel therapies. In mouse models, caloric restriction is capable of curing fatty liver disease [105].

The function of ERRs as master regulators for metabolism made them interesting targets for the treatment of T2D, as activating ERRs has the potential to improve overall mitochondrial respiratory function and suppress hepatic glucose output. Earlier studies, tethered with the elucidation of LBD structures, have focused on developing agonists or antagonists. These studies show that ERRs are constitutively active and identified several estrogen-related hydrophilic molecules that can bind and block the establishment of active conformations. These molecules such as the diethylstilbestrol (DES) and 4-hydroxytamoxifen (4-OHT) have been described as antagonists for ERRs, where DES binds to all three ERRs, and 4-OHT does not bind to ERRα [106, 107].

Due to the lack of endogenous ligand, XCT-790 was identified as a potent inverse agonist for ERRα and is used in many studies as inhibitors of ERR functions [108]. Using the NIH compound library in a couple high throughput screening studies, it was found that several pesticides contain ERRβ genes promoting activities, and these compounds may act as potential "ligands" for ERRs [109, 110]. The activity of ERRα has been reported to be antagonized by the organochlorine pesticides chlordane and toxaphene [111, 112]. Screening approaches also identified small molecules with the ability to alter ERR transcriptional activity. An example is the discovery of compound 11 that potently inhibits ERRα's transcriptional activity by preventing binding of ERRα to PGC-1α and suppressing the proliferation of different cancer cell lines [113].

Troglitazone also interferes with binding of ERRα and γ to PGC-1α. Troglitazone was recently discovered to be an inverse agonist for ERRα and γ [114]. Troglitazone is an FDA approved therapy for T2D. In hepatocytes, troglitazone inhibits oleic acid induced liquid buildup. Thus, activity of troglitazone towards ERRα likely plays a role in this effect. In addition, pharmacological inhibition of either ERRα or ERRγ has led to improved insulin response and better tolerance to diet induced metabolic changes [79, 80].

Beyond identification of ligand-like molecules that can serve as either antagonist or agonist for ERR, effort was put into blocking its binding to DNA. Pyrrole-imidazole (Py-Im) polyamides are a class of synthetic ligands for the sequence-specific recognition in double-helical DNA minor groove [84]. Polyamides targeted at the ERRE (ERR-PA) were designed to block binding of ERR onto the promoters of genes regulated by it. An *in vitro* study showed that there was over a 50% reduction in basal and maximal respiration with 0.2 μM ERR-PA treatment and around 70% reduction with 1 μM, emphasizing the dose dependency of the polyamide molecule [84]. ERR-PA was highly effective at reducing liver steatosis in multiple NAFLD models, including one with deletion of *Pten*, the negative regulator of insulin signal; a HFD model, which induces lipid transport into the liver; and a HCD model that induces *de novo* lipogenesis. ERR-PA also reversed the NASH phenotypes observed in the mice where NAFLD/NASH is developed due to loss of hepatic *Pten*. This evidence suggest that inhibiting ERR activity can serve as a viable approach to treat NAFLD/NASH development.

TGs are the primary content induced in NAFLD/NASH. TGs are synthesized via the glycerolipid biosynthesis pathway, where Glycerol-3-phosphate (G3P) and acyl-CoA is converted to LPA with the help of GPAT enzyme activity followed by incorporation into DAG and TG. Enzymes catalyzing the steps in this biosynthesis are subjected to regulations by ERR and other nuclear transcriptional factors. *Gpat1*-null mice were found to have lower triacylglycerol and DAG concentrations and were protected from the HFD-induced insulin resistance, which was attributed to lower DAG-mediated PKCε activation [115]. Mice lacking GPAT3 expression had increased liver size with dysregulated cholesterol metabolism, implying that *Gpat3* plays a crucial role in regulating energy, glucose, and lipid levels [116]. GPAT4 is the major isoform in the liver and mammary gland [117]. Recent work has identified GPAT4 as a direct transcriptional target for ERRα and could be responsible for ERRα regulated NAFLD development [84].

8. Conclusion

ERRs are a family of orphan NRs that do not have a known endogenous ligand. Of the three isoforms of ERRs (ERRα, ERRβ, and ERRγ), ERRα and ERRγ are involved in the transcriptional regulation of mitochondrial metabolism and integrity, OXPHOS, glucose and lipid metabolism metabolism, while ERRβ plays a role in embryonic development. The transcriptional activity of ERRs requires binding with coactivator PGC-1α. ERRs share overlapping functions with PGC-1α regulated transcriptional networks and are subjected to the factors that regulate PGC-1α. In addition, ERRs are regulated post-translationally by upstream signal that also include the insulin regulated PI3K/AKT signaling pathways. In recent years, a major development in the cellular functions regulated by ERRs is the discovery of lipogenesis and glycerolipid biosynthesis regulation by ERR. These functions of ERRs allow them to play major roles in NAFLD/NASH development. Pharmacologically, significant efforts have been put forth to identify ligands for ERRs and these studies identified several agonists and antagonists for ERRs that can be further developed for future therapeutical efforts. Notably, DBD antagonists are also being developed and shown strong promise at targeting NAFLD. This review provides a brief and comprehensive view for the transcriptional network regulated by ERRs and their functions in NAFLD and potential therapeutical developments targeted at ERRs.

Acknowledgements

Dr. Stiles would like to acknowledge funding from NIDDK DK131492.

Conflict of interest

The authors declare no conflict of interest.

Acronyms and abbreviations

ERR	estrogen related receptor
NR	nuclear receptor
OXPHOS	oxidative phosphorylation
TCA	tricarboxylic acid
T2D	type II diabetes
IR	insulin resistance
NAFLD	non-alcoholic liver disease
NASH	non-alcoholic steatohepatitis
ER	estrogen receptor
DBD	DNA-binding domain
ERRE	estrogen related response element
AF-1	activation-function-1
LBD	ligand binding domain
SRC-1	steroid receptor coactivator 1
ERE	estrogen response element
GAPDH	glyceraldehyde dehydrogenase
PPARγ	peroxisomal proliferation activated receptor γ
PGC-1	coactivator-1
mEFs	mouse embryonic fibroblasts
α-KG	α-ketoglutarate
MCAD	medium chain acyl-CoA decarboxylase
iPS	immortalized pluripotent stem cells
OSN	OCT4-SOX2-Nanog
LIF	leukemia inhibitory factor
NRF	nuclear respiratory factor
AMPK	AMP activated kinase
EGF	epidermal growth factor
PTEN	phosphatase and tensin homolog deleted on chromosome 10
OCR	oxygen consumption
LEF-1	lymphoid enhanced-binding factor-1
Fasn	fatty acid synthase
ACC	acetyl-CoA carboxylase
TG	triglyceride
LPA	lysophosphatidic acid
PA	phosphatidic acid
DAG	diacylglycerol
HFD	high fat diet
HCD	high carbohydrate diet
PI3K	phosphoinositide 3-kinase
mTOR	mammalian target of rapamycin
cyclic AMP (cAMP)	response element binding protein (CREB)
DES	diethylstilbestrol
4-OHT	4-hydroxytamoxifen
Py-Im	pyrole-imidazole
G3P	glycerol-3-phosphate

Author details

Brittney Hua[1], Ielyzaveta Slarve[1], Aditi A. Datta[1], Chenxi Xu[1], Chien-yu Chen[1] and Bangyan L. Stiles[1,2]*

1 Pharmacology and Pharmaceutical Sciences, School of Pharmacy, University of Southern California, United States

2 Department of Pathology, Keck School of Medicine, University of Southern California, United States

*Address all correspondence to: bstiles@usc.edu

References

[1] Knutti D, Kralli A. PGC-1, a versatile coactivator. Trends in Endocrinology and Metabolism. 2001;**12**(8):360-365. DOI: 10.1016/S1043-2760(01)00457-X

[2] Deblois G, Giguère V. Functional and physiological genomics of estrogen-related receptors (ERRs) in health and disease. Biochimica et Biophysica Acta (BBA) - Molecular Basis of Disease. 2011;**1812**(8):1032-1040. DOI: 10.1016/j.bbadis.2010.12.009

[3] Hummasti S, Tontonoz P. Adopting new orphans into the family of metabolic regulators. Molecular Endocrinology. 2008;**22**(8):1743-1753. DOI: 10.1210/me.2007-0566

[4] Scarpulla RC. Nuclear control of respiratory gene expression in mammalian cells. Journal of Cellular Biochemistry. 2006;**97**(4):673-683. DOI: 10.1002/jcb.20743

[5] Vercauteren K, Gleyzer N, Scarpulla RC. Short hairpin RNA-mediated silencing of PRC (PGC-1-related coactivator) results in a severe respiratory chain deficiency associated with the proliferation of aberrant mitochondria. The Journal of Biological Chemistry. 2009;**284**(4):2307-2319. DOI: 10.1074/jbc.M806434200

[6] Villena JA, Kralli A. ERRα: A metabolic function for the oldest orphan. Trends in Endocrinology and Metabolism. 2008;**19**(8):269-276. DOI: 10.1016/j.tem.2008.07.005

[7] Giguère V, Yang N, Segui P, Evans RM. Identification of a new class of steroid hormone receptors. Nature. 1988;**331**(6151):91-94. DOI: 10.1038/331091a0

[8] Misawa A, Inoue S. Estrogen-related receptors in breast cancer and prostate cancer. Frontiers in Endocrinology (Lausanne). 2015;**6**:1-7. DOI: 10.3389/fendo.2015.00083

[9] Laudet V, Hänni C, Coll J, Catzeflis F, Stéhelin D. Evolution of the nuclear receptor gene superfamily. EMBO Journal. 1992;**11**(3):1003-1013. DOI: 10.1002/j.1460-2075.1992.tb05139.x

[10] Sladek R, Bader JA, Giguère V. The orphan nuclear receptor estrogen-related receptor alpha is a transcriptional regulator of the human medium-chain acyl coenzyme A dehydrogenase gene. Molecular and Cellular Biology. 1997;**17**(9):5400-5409. DOI: 10.1128/mcb.17.9.5400

[11] Wärnmark A, Treuter E, Wright APH, Gustafsson JÅ. Activation functions 1 and 2 of nuclear receptors: Molecular strategies for transcriptional activation. Molecular Endocrinology. 2003;**17**(10):1901-1909. DOI: 10.1210/me.2002-0384

[12] Handa RJ, Larco DO, Wu TJ. Steroid hormone action in health and disease. Reference Module in Biomedical Sciences. Published online. 2014:1-11. DOI: 10.1016/b978-0-12-801238-3.00099-4

[13] Kraus RJ, Ariazi EA, Farrell ML, Mertz JE. Estrogen-related receptor α1 actively antagonizes estrogen receptor-regulated transcription in MCF-7 mammary cells. The Journal of Biological Chemistry. 2002;**277**(27):24826-24834. DOI: 10.1074/jbc.M202952200

[14] Ricketson D, Hostick U, Fang L, Yamamoto KR, Darimont BD. A conformational switch in the ligand-binding domain regulates the dependence of the glucocorticoid receptor on Hsp90. Journal of Molecular Biology. 2007;**368**(3):729-741. DOI: 10.1016/j.jmb.2007.02.057

[15] Deblois G, Hall JA, Perry MC, et al. Genome-wide identification of direct target genes implicates estrogen-related receptor α as a determinant of breast cancer heterogeneity. Cancer Research. 2009;**69**(15):6149-6157. DOI: 10.1158/0008-5472.CAN-09-1251

[16] Greschik H, Wurtz JM, Sanglier S, et al. Structural and functional evidence for ligand-independent transcriptional activation by the estrogen-related receptor 3. Molecular Cell. 2002;**9**(2):303-313. DOI: 10.1016/S1097-2765(02)00444-6

[17] Kallen J, Schlaeppi JM, Bitsch F, et al. Evidence for ligand-independent transcriptional activation of the human estrogen-related receptor α (ERRα): Crystal structure of ERRα ligand binding domain in complex with peroxisome proliferator-activated receptor coactivator-1α. The Journal of Biological Chemistry. 2004;**279**(47):49330-49337. DOI: 10.1074/jbc.M407999200

[18] Yao B, Zhang S, Wei Y, et al. Structural insights into the specificity of ligand binding and coactivator assembly by estrogen-related receptor β. Journal of Molecular Biology. 2020;**432**(19):5460-5472. DOI: 10.1016/j.jmb.2020.08.007

[19] Misu H, Takamura T, Matsuzawa N, et al. Genes involved in oxidative phosphorylation are coordinately upregulated with fasting hyperglycaemia in livers of patients with type 2 diabetes. Diabetologia. 2007;**50**(2):268-277. DOI: 10.1007/s00125-006-0489-8

[20] Mootha VK, Handschin C, Arlow D, et al. Errα and Gabpa/b specify PGC-1α-dependent oxidative phosphorylation gene expression that is altered in diabetic muscle. Proceedings of the National Academy of Sciences of the United States of America. 2004;**101**(17):6570-6575. DOI: 10.1073/pnas.0401401101

[21] Schreiber SN, Emter R, Hock MB, et al. The estrogen-related receptor alpha (ERRalpha) functions in PPARgamma coactivator 1alpha (PGC-1alpha)-induced mitochondrial biogenesis. Proceedings of the National Academy of Sciences of the United States of America. 2004;**101**(17):6472-6477. DOI: 10.1073/pnas.0308686101

[22] Huss JM, Torra IP, Staels B, Giguère V, Kelly DP. Estrogen-related receptor α; directs peroxisome proliferator-activated receptor α; signaling in the transcriptional control of energy metabolism in cardiac and skeletal muscle. Molecular and Cellular Biology. 2004;**24**(20):9079-9091. DOI: 10.1128/MCB.24.20.9079-9091.2004

[23] Madhu Krishna B, Chaudhary S, Mishra DR, et al. Estrogen receptor α dependent regulation of estrogen related receptor β and its role in cell cycle in breast cancer. BMC Cancer. 2018;**18**(1):1-15. DOI: 10.1186/s12885-018-4528-x

[24] Zhang Z, Chen K, Shih JC, Teng CT. Estrogen-related receptors-stimulated monoamine oxidase B promoter activity is down-regulated by estrogen receptors. Molecular Endocrinology. 2006;**20**(7):1547-1561. DOI: 10.1210/me.2005-0252

[25] Lu D, Kiriyama Y, Lee KY, Giguère V. Transcriptional regulation of the estrogen-inducible pS2 breast cancer marker gene by the ERR family of orphan nuclear receptors. Cancer Research. 2001;**61**(18):6755-6761

[26] Luo J, Sladek R, Carrier J, Bader J-A, Richard D, Giguère V. reduced fat mass in mice lacking orphan nuclear receptor estrogen-related receptor α. Molecular and Cellular Biology. 2003;**23**(22):7947-7956. DOI: 10.1128/mcb.23.22.7947-7956.2003

[27] Audet-Walsh É, Giguére V. The multiple universes of estrogen-related

receptor α and γ in metabolic control and related diseases. Acta Pharmacologica Sinica. 2015;**36**(1):51-61. DOI: 10.1038/aps.2014.121

[28] Cai Q, Lin T, Kamarajugadda S, Lu J. Regulation of glycolysis and the Warburg effect by estrogen-related receptors. Oncogene. 2013;**32**(16):2079-2086. DOI: 10.1038/onc.2012.221

[29] Huss JM, Garbacz WG, Xie W. Constitutive activities of estrogen-related receptors: Transcriptional regulation of metabolism by the ERR pathways in health and disease. Biochimica et Biophysica Acta (BBA) - Molecular Basis of Disease. 2015;**1852**(9):1912-1927. DOI: 10.1016/j.bbadis.2015.06.016

[30] Rangwala SM, Li X, Lindsley L, et al. Estrogen-related receptor α is essential for the expression of antioxidant protection genes and mitochondrial function. Biochemical and Biophysical Research Communications. 2007;**357**(1):231-236. DOI: 10.1016/j.bbrc.2007.03.126

[31] Dufour CR, Wilson BJ, Huss JM, et al. Genome-wide orchestration of cardiac functions by the orphan nuclear receptors ERRα and γ. Cell Metabolism. 2007;**5**(5):345-356. DOI: 10.1016/j.cmet.2007.03.007

[32] Wang T, McDonald C, Petrenko NB, et al. Estrogen-related receptor α (ERRα) and ERRγ are essential coordinators of cardiac metabolism and function. Molecular and Cellular Biology. 2015;**35**(7):1281-1298. DOI: 10.1128/mcb.01156-14

[33] Herzog B, Cardenas J, Hall RK, et al. Estrogen-related receptor α is a repressor of phosphoenolpyruvate carboxykinase gene transcription. The Journal of Biological Chemistry. 2006;**281**(1):99-106. DOI: 10.1074/jbc.M509276200

[34] Kim DK, Ryu D, Koh M, et al. Orphan nuclear receptor estrogen-related receptor γ(ERRγ) is key regulator of hepatic gluconeogenesis. The Journal of Biological Chemistry. 2012;**287**(26):21628-21639. DOI: 10.1074/jbc.M111.315168

[35] Kwon DH, Eom GH, Kee HJ, et al. Estrogen-related receptor gamma induces cardiac hypertrophy by activating GATA4. Journal of Molecular and Cellular Cardiology. 2013;**65**:88-97. DOI: 10.1016/j.yjmcc.2013.09.011

[36] Ariazi EA, Clark GM, Mertz JE. Estrogen-related receptor α and estrogen-related receptor γ associate with unfavorable and favorable biomarkers, respectively, in human breast cancer. Cancer Research. 2002;**62**(22):6510-6518

[37] Kang MH, Choi H, Oshima M, et al. Estrogen-related receptor gamma functions as a tumor suppressor in gastric cancer. Nature Communications. 2018;**9**(1):1-13. DOI: 10.1038/s41467-018-04244-2

[38] Fox SN, McMeekin LJ, Savage CH, et al. Estrogen-related receptor gamma regulates mitochondrial and synaptic genes and modulates vulnerability to synucleinopathy. NPJ Parkinson's Disease. 2022;**8**(1):106. DOI: 10.1038/s41531-022-00369-w

[39] Festuccia N, Osorno R, Halbritter F, et al. Esrrb is a direct Nanog target gene that can substitute for Nanog function in pluripotent cells. Cell Stem Cell. 2012;**11**(4):477-490. DOI: 10.1016/j.stem.2012.08.002

[40] Hutchins AP, Choo SH, Mistri TK, et al. Co-motif discovery identifies an esrrb-Sox2-DNA ternary complex as a mediator of transcriptional differences between mouse embryonic and epiblast stem cells. Stem Cells. 2013;**31**(2):269-281. DOI: 10.1002/stem.1279

[41] van den Berg DLC, Zhang W, Yates A, et al. Estrogen-related receptor beta interacts with Oct4 to positively regulate nanog gene expression. Molecular and Cellular Biology. 2008;**28**(19):5986-5995. DOI: 10.1128/mcb.00301-08

[42] Feng B, Jiang J, Kraus P, et al. Reprogramming of fibroblasts into induced pluripotent stem cells with orphan nuclear receptor Esrrb. Nature Cell Biology. 2009;**11**(2):197-203. DOI: 10.1038/ncb1827

[43] Chen X, Xu H, Yuan P, et al. Integration of external signaling pathways with the core transcriptional network in embryonic stem cells. Cell. 2008;**133**(6):1106-1117. DOI: 10.1016/j.cell.2008.04.043

[44] Charest-Marcotte A, Dufour CR, Wilson BJ, et al. The homeobox protein Prox1 is a negative modulator of ERRα/PGC-1α bioenergetic functions. Genes & Development. 2010;**24**(6):537-542. DOI: 10.1101/gad.1871610

[45] Huang D, Wang L, Duan J, et al. LIF-Activated Jak signaling determines Esrrb expression during late-stage reprogramming. Biology Open. 2018;7(1):2-8. DOI: 10.1242/bio.029264

[46] Katano M, Ema M, Nakachi Y, et al. Forced expression of Nanog or Esrrb preserves the ESC status in the absence of nucleostemin expression. Stem Cells. 2015;**33**(4):1089-1101. DOI: 10.1002/stem.1918

[47] Martello G, Sugimoto T, Diamanti E, et al. Esrrb is a pivotal target of the Gsk3/Tcf3 axis regulating embryonic stem cell self-renewal. Cell Stem Cell. 2012;**11**(4):491-504. DOI: 10.1016/j.stem.2012.06.008

[48] Percharde M, Lavial F, Ng JH, et al. Ncoa3 functions as an essential Esrrb coactivator to sustain embryonic stem cell self-renewal and reprogramming. Genes & Development. 2012;**26**(20):2286-2298. DOI: 10.1101/gad.195545.112

[49] Divekar SD, Tiek DM, Fernandez A, Riggins RB. Estrogen-related receptor β (ERRβ) - renaissance receptor or receptor renaissance? Nuclear Receptor Signaling. 2016;**14**:e002. DOI: 10.1621/nrs.14002

[50] Luo J, Sladek R, Bader JA, Matthyssen A, Rossant J, Giguère V. Placental abnormalities in mouse embryos lacking the orphan nuclear receptor ERR-β. Nature. 1997;**388**(6644):778-782. DOI: 10.1038/42022

[51] Auld KL, Berasi SP, Liu Y, et al. Estrogen-related receptor α regulates osteoblast differentiation via Wnt/β-catenin signaling. Journal of Molecular Endocrinology. 2012;**48**(2):177-191. DOI: 10.1530/JME-11-0140

[52] Delhon I, Gutzwiller S, Morvan F, et al. Absence of estrogen receptor-related-α increases osteoblastic differentiation and cancellous bone mineral density. Endocrinology. 2009;**150**(10):4463-4472. DOI: 10.1210/en.2009-0121

[53] Mitsunaga K, Araki K, Mizusaki H, et al. Loss of PGC-specific expression of the orphan nuclear receptor ERR-β results in reduction of germ cell number in mouse embryos. Mechanisms of Development. 2004;**121**(3):237-246. DOI: 10.1016/j.mod.2004.01.006

[54] Kida YS, Kawamura T, Wei Z, et al. ERRs mediate a metabolic switch required for somatic cell reprogramming to pluripotency. Cell Stem Cell. 2015;**16**(5):547-555. DOI: 10.1016/j.stem.2015.03.001

[55] Cunningham KF, Beeson GC, Beeson CC, McDermott PJ. Increased expression of estrogen-related

receptor β during adaptation of adult cardiomyocytes to sustained hypoxia. American Journal of Cardiovascular Disease 2016;6(2):46-54. Available from: http://www.ncbi.nlm.nih.gov/pubmed/27335690%0Ahttp://www.pubmedcentral.nih.gov/articlerender.fcgi?artid=PMC4913214

[56] Rowe GC, Jiang A, Arany Z. PGC-1 coactivators in cardiac development and disease. Circulation Research. 2010;**107**(7):825-838. DOI: 10.1161/CIRCRESAHA.110.223818

[57] Huss JM, Kopp RP, Kelly DP. Peroxisome proliferator-activated receptor coactivator-1α (PGC-1α) coactivates the cardiac-enriched nuclear receptors estrogen-related receptor-α and -γ: Identification of novel Leucine-rich interaction motif within PGC-1α. The Journal of Biological Chemistry. 2002;**277**(43):40265-40274. DOI: 10.1074/jbc.M206324200

[58] Puigserver P, Wu Z, Park CW, Graves R, Wright M, Spiegelman BM. A cold-inducible coactivator of nuclear receptors linked to adaptive thermogenesis. Cell. 1998;**92**(6):829-839. DOI: 10.1016/S0092-8674(00)81410-5

[59] Gaillard S, Grasfeder LL, Haeffele CL, et al. Receptor-selective coactivators as tools to define the biology of specific receptor-coactivator pairs. Molecular Cell. 2006;**24**(5):797-803. DOI: 10.1016/j.molcel.2006.10.012

[60] Schreiber SN, Knutti D, Brogli K, Uhlmann T, Kralli A. The transcriptional coactivator PGC-1 regulates the expression and activity of the orphan nuclear receptor estrogen-related receptor α (ERRα). The Journal of Biological Chemistry. 2003;**278**(11):9013-9018. DOI: 10.1074/jbc.M212923200

[61] Laganière J, Tremblay GB, Dufour CR, Giroux S, Rousseau F, Giguère V. A polymorphic autoregulatory hormone response element in the human estrogen-related receptor α (ERRα) promoter dictates peroxisome proliferator-activated receptor γ coactivator-1α control of ERRα expression. The Journal of Biological Chemistry. 2004;**279**(18):18504-18510. DOI: 10.1074/jbc.M313543200

[62] Devarakonda S, Gupta K, Chalmers MJ, et al. Disorder-to-order transition underlies the structural basis for the assembly of a transcriptionally active PGC-1α/ERRγ complex. Proceedings of the National Academy of Sciences of the United States of America. 2011;**108**(46):18678-18683. DOI: 10.1073/pnas.1113813108

[63] Puigserver P, Adelmant G, Wu Z, et al. Activation of PPARγ coactivator-1 through transcription factor docking. Science (80-). 1999;**286**(5443):1368-1371. DOI:10.1126/science.286.5443.1368

[64] Jäer S, Handschin C, St-Pierre J, Spiegelman BM. AMP-activated protein kinase (AMPK) action in skeletal muscle via direct phosphorylation of PGC-1α. Proceedings of the National Academy of Sciences of the United States of America. 2007;**104**(29):12017-12022. DOI: 10.1073/pnas.0705070104

[65] Li X, Monks B, Ge Q, Birnbaum MJ. Akt/PKB regulates hepatic metabolism by directly inhibiting PGC-1α transcription coactivator. Nature. 2007;**447**(7147):1012-1016. DOI: 10.1038/nature05861

[66] Lustig Y, Ruas JL, Estall JL, et al. Separation of the gluconeogenic and mitochondrial functions of pgc-1α through s6 kinase. Genes & Development. 2011;**25**(12):1232-1244. DOI: 10.1101/gad.2054711

[67] Gerhart-Hines Z, Rodgers JT, Bare O, et al. Metabolic control of muscle mitochondrial function and fatty acid oxidation through SIRT1/PGC-1α. The EMBO Journal. 2007;**26**(7):1913-1923. DOI: 10.1038/sj.emboj.7601633

[68] Luo X, Liao C, Quan J, et al. Posttranslational regulation of PGC-1α and its implication in cancer metabolism. International Journal of Cancer. 2019;**145**(6):1475-1483. DOI: 10.1002/ijc.32253

[69] Barry JB, Giguère V. Epidermal growth factor-induced signaling in breast cancer cells results in selective target gene activation by orphan nuclear receptor estrogen-related receptor α. Cancer Research. 2005;**65**(14):6120-6129. DOI: 10.1158/0008-5472.CAN-05-0922

[70] Ariazi EA, Kraus RJ, Farrell ML, Jordan VC, Mertz JE. Estrogen-related receptor α1 transcriptional activities are regulated in part via the ErbB2/HER2 signaling pathway. Molecular Cancer Research. 2007;**5**(1):71-85. DOI: 10.1158/1541-7786.MCR-06-0227

[71] Wallace DC. Mitochondria and cancer: Warburg addressed. Cold Spring Harbor Symposia on Quantitative Biology. 2005;**70**:363-374. DOI: 10.1101/sqb.2005.70.035

[72] Li Y, He L, Zeng N, et al. Phosphatase and tensin homolog deleted on chromosome 10 (PTEN) signaling regulates mitochondrial biogenesis and respiration via estrogen-related receptor α (ERRα). The Journal of Biological Chemistry. 2013;**288**(35):25007-25024. DOI: 10.1074/jbc.M113.450353

[73] Cerniglia GJ, Dey S, Gallagher-Colombo SM, et al. The PI3K/Akt pathway regulates oxygen metabolism via pyruvate dehydrogenase (PDH)-E1α phosphorylation. Molecular Cancer Therapeutics. 2015;**14**(8):1928-1938. DOI: 10.1158/1535-7163.MCT-14-0888

[74] Tremblay AM, Wilson BJ, Yang XJ, Giguère V. Phosphorylation-dependent sumoylation regulates estrogen-related receptor-β and -γ transcriptional activity through a synergy control motif. Molecular Endocrinology. 2008;**22**(3):570-584. DOI: 10.1210/me.2007-0357

[75] Dwyer MA, Joseph JD, Wade HE, et al. WNT11 expression is induced by estrogen-related receptor α and β-catenin and acts in an autocrine manner to increase cancer cell migration. Cancer Research. 2010;**70**(22):9298-9308. DOI: 10.1158/0008-5472.CAN-10-0226

[76] Alaynick WA, Kondo RP, Xie W, et al. ERRγ directs and maintains the transition to oxidative metabolism in the postnatal heart. Cell Metabolism. 2007;**6**(1):13-24. DOI: 10.1016/j.cmet.2007.06.007

[77] Huss JM, Imahashi K-i, Dufour CR, et al. The nuclear receptor ERRα is required for the bioenergetic and functional adaptation to cardiac pressure overload. Cell Metabolism. 2007;**6**(1):25-37. DOI: 10.1016/j.cmet.2007.06.005

[78] Villena JA, Hock MB, Chang WY, Barcas JE, Giguère V, Kralli A. Orphan nuclear receptor estrogen-related receptor α is essential for adaptive themogenesis. Proceedings of the National Academy of Sciences of the United States of America. 2007;**104**(4):1418-1423. DOI: 10.1073/pnas.0607696104

[79] Kim DK, Kim JR, Koh M, et al. Estrogen-related receptor γ (ERRγ) is a novel transcriptional regulator of phosphatidic acid phosphatase, LIPIN1, and inhibits hepatic insulin signaling. The Journal of Biological Chemistry. 2011;**286**(44):38035-38042. DOI: 10.1074/jbc.M111.250613

[80] Patch RJ, Searle LL, Kim AJ, et al. Identification of diaryl ether-based ligands for estrogen-related receptor α as potential antidiabetic agents. Journal of Medicinal Chemistry. 2011;**54**(3):788-808. DOI: 10.1021/jm101063h

[81] Ijichi N, Ikeda K, Horie-Inoue K, Yagi K, Okazaki Y, Inoue S. Estrogen-related receptor α modulates the expression of adipogenesis-related genes during adipocyte differentiation. Biochemical and Biophysical Research Communications. 2007;**358**(3):813-818. DOI: 10.1016/j.bbrc.2007.04.209

[82] Ju D, He J, Zhao L, Zheng X, Yang G. Estrogen related receptor α-induced adipogenesis is PGC-1β-dependent. Molecular Biology Reports. 2012;**39**(3):3343-3354. DOI: 10.1007/s11033-011-1104-8

[83] Chaveroux C, Eichner LJ, Dufour CR, et al. Molecular and genetic crosstalks between mTOR and ERRα are key determinants of rapamycin-induced nonalcoholic fatty liver. Cell Metabolism. 2013;**17**(4):586-598. DOI: 10.1016/j.cmet.2013.03.003

[84] Yu CC, Li Y, Zeng N, et al. Inhibition of estrogen-related receptor α blocks liver steatosis and steatohepatitis and attenuates triglyceride biosynthesis. The American Journal of Pathology. 2021;**191**(7):1240-1254. DOI: 10.1016/j.ajpath.2021.04.007

[85] Karasawa K, Tanigawa K, Harada A, Yamashita A. Transcriptional Regulation of Acyl-CoA: Glycerol-sn-3-Phosphate Acyltransferases. International Journal of Molecular Sciences. 2019;**20**(4):964. DOI: 10.3390/ijms20040964

[86] Jou J, Choi SS, Diehl AM. Mechanisms of disease progression in nonalcoholic fatty liver disease. Seminars in Liver Disease. 2008;**28**(4):370-379. DOI: 10.1055/s-0028-1091981

[87] Schattenberg JM, Schuppan D. Nonalcoholic steatohepatitis: The therapeutic challenge of a global epidemic. Current Opinion in Lipidology. 2011;**22**(6):479-488. DOI: 10.1097/MOL.0b013e32834c7cfc

[88] Jeon S, Carr R. Alcohol effects on hepatic lipid metabolism. Journal of Lipid Research. 2020;**61**(4):470-479. DOI: 10.1194/jlr.R119000547

[89] Lackner C, Tiniakos D. Fibrosis and alcohol-related liver disease. Journal of Hepatology. 2019;**70**(2):294-304. DOI: 10.1016/j.jhep.2018.12.003

[90] Rosny E de, Groot A de, Jullian-Binard C, et al. DHR51, the Drosophila melanogaster homologue of the human photoreceptor cell-specific nuclear receptor, is a thiolate heme-binding protein. Biochemistry. 2008;**47**(50):13252-13260. DOI: 10.1021/bi801691b

[91] Brown MS, Goldstein JL. Selective versus total insulin resistance: A pathogenic paradox. Cell Metabolism. 2008;**7**(2):95-96. DOI: 10.1016/j.cmet.2007.12.009

[92] Yang J, Nie J, Ma X, Wei Y, Peng Y, Wei X. Targeting PI3K in cancer: Mechanisms and advances in clinical trials. Molecular Cancer. 2019;**18**(1):26. DOI: 10.1186/s12943-019-0954-x

[93] Stiles B, Wang Y, Stahl A, et al. Liver-specific deletion of negative regulator Pten results in fatty liver and insulin hypersensitivity [corrected]. Proceedings of the National Academy of Sciences of the United States of America. 2004;**101**(7):2082-2087. DOI: 10.1073/pnas.0308617100

[94] Chen J, Debebe A, Zeng N, et al. Transformation of SOX9+ cells by Pten deletion synergizes with steatotic liver injury to drive development of hepatocellular and cholangiocarcinoma. Scientific Reports. 2021;**11**(1):11823. DOI: 10.1038/s41598-021-90958-1

[95] Debebe A, Medina V, Chen CY, et al. Wnt/β-catenin activation and

macrophage induction during liver cancer development following steatosis. Oncogene. 2017;**36**(43):6020-6029. DOI: 10.1038/onc.2017.207

[96] Galicia VA, He L, Dang H, et al. Expansion of hepatic tumor progenitor cells in Pten-null mice requires liver injury and is reversed by loss of AKT2. Gastroenterology. 2010;**139**(6):2170-2182. DOI: 10.1053/j.gastro.2010.09.002

[97] He L, Hou X, Kanel G, et al. The critical role of AKT2 in hepatic steatosis induced by PTEN loss. American Journal of Pathology. 2010;**176**(5):2302-2308. DOI: 10.2353/ajpath.2010.090931

[98] Li C, Li Y, He L, et al. PI3K/AKT signaling regulates bioenergetics in immortalized hepatocytes. Free Radical Biology and Medicine. 2013;**60**:29-40. DOI: 10.1016/j.freeradbiomed.2013.01.013

[99] Zhang X, Odom DT, Koo SH, et al. Genome-wide analysis of cAMP-response element binding protein occupancy, phosphorylation, and target gene activation in human tissues. Proceedings of the National Academy of Sciences of the United States of America. 2005;**102**(12):4459-4464. DOI: 10.1073/pnas.0501076102

[100] Herzig S, Hedrick S, Morantte I, Koo SH, Galimi F, Montminy M. CREB controls hepatic lipid metabolism through nuclear hormone receptor PPAR-gamma. Nature. 2003;**426**(6963):190-193. DOI: 10.1038/nature02110

[101] Herzig S, Long F, Jhala US, et al. CREB regulates hepatic gluconeogenesis through the coactivator PGC-1. Nature. 2001;**413**(6852):179-183. DOI: 10.1038/35093131

[102] Erion DM, Ignatova ID, Yonemitsu S, et al. Prevention of hepatic steatosis and hepatic insulin resistance by knockdown of cAMP response element-binding protein. Cell Metabolism. 2009;**10**(6):499-506. DOI: 10.1016/j.cmet.2009.10.007

[103] B'chir W, Dufour CR, Ouellet C, et al. Divergent Role of Estrogen-Related Receptor α in Lipid- and Fasting-Induced Hepatic Steatosis in Mice. Endocrinology. 2018;**159**(5):2153-2164. DOI: 10.1210/en.2018-00115

[104] Brar G, Tsukamoto H. Alcoholic and non-alcoholic steatohepatitis: Global perspective and emerging science. Journal of Gastroenterology. 2019;**54**(3):218-225. DOI: 10.1007/s00535-018-01542-w

[105] Mazhar K. The Future of Nonalcoholic Fatty Liver Disease Treatment. Medical Clinics of North America. 2019;**103**(1):57-69. DOI: 10.1016/j.mcna.2018.08.005

[106] Tremblay GB, Bergeron D, Giguere V. 4-Hydroxytamoxifen is an isoform-specific inhibitor of orphan estrogen-receptor-related (ERR) nuclear receptors beta and gamma. Endocrinology. 2001;**142**(10):4572-4575. DOI: 10.1210/endo.142.10.8528

[107] Greschik H, Flaig R, Renaud JP, Moras D. Structural basis for the deactivation of the estrogen-related receptor gamma by diethylstilbestrol or 4-hydroxytamoxifen and determinants of selectivity. Journal of Biological Chemistry. 2004;**279**(32):33639-33646. DOI: 10.1074/jbc.M402195200

[108] Busch BB, Stevens WC Jr, Martin R, et al. Identification of a selective inverse agonist for the orphan nuclear receptor estrogen-related receptor alpha. Journal of Medicinal Chemistry. 2004;**47**(23):5593-5596. DOI: 10.1021/jm049334f

[109] Lynch C, Zhao J, Sakamuru S, et al. Identification of Compounds That

Inhibit Estrogen-Related Receptor Alpha Signaling Using High-Throughput Screening Assays. Molecules. 2019;**24**(5):841. DOI: 10.3390/molecules24050841

[110] Lynch C, Zhao J, Xia M. Cell-Based Assays to Identify ERR and ERR/PGC Modulators. Methods of Molecular Biology. 2022;**2474**:3-9. DOI: 10.1007/978-1-0716-2213-1_1

[111] Chen S, Zhou D, Yang C, Sherman M. Molecular basis for the constitutive activity of estrogen-related receptor alpha-1. Journal of Biological Chemistry. 2001;**276**(30):28465-28470. DOI: 10.1074/jbc.M102638200

[112] Yang C, Chen S. Two organochlorine pesticides, toxaphene and chlordane, are antagonists for estrogen-related receptor α-1 orphan receptor1. Cancer Research. 1999;**59**(18):4519-4524

[113] Du Y, Song L, Zhang L, et al. The discovery of novel, potent ERR-alpha inverse agonists for the treatment of triple negative breast cancer. European Journal of Medicinal Chemistry. 2017;**136**:457-467

[114] Wang Y, Fang F, Wong CW. Troglitazone is an estrogen-related receptor alpha and gamma inverse agonist. Biochemical Pharmacology. 2010;**80**(1):80-85. DOI: 10.1016/j.bcp.2010.03.013

[115] Neschen S, Morino K, Hammond LE, et al. Prevention of hepatic steatosis and hepatic insulin resistance in mitochondrial acyl-CoA:glycerol-sn-3-phosphate acyltransferase 1 knockout mice. Cell Metabolism. 2005;**2**(1):55-65. DOI: 10.1016/j.cmet.2005.06.006

[116] Cao J, Perez S, Goodwin B, et al. Mice deleted for GPAT3 have reduced GPAT activity in white adipose tissue and altered energy and cholesterol homeostasis in diet-induced obesity. American Journal of Physiology-Endocrinology and Metabolism. 2014;**306**(10):E1176-1187. DOI: 10.1152/ajpendo.00666.2013

[117] Nagle CA, Vergnes L, Dejong H, Wang S, Lewin TM, Reue K, et al. Identification of a novel sn-glycerol-3-phosphate acyltransferase isoform, GPAT4, as the enzyme deficient in Agpat6-/- mice. Journal of Lipid Research. 2008;**49**(4):823-831. DOI: 10.1194/jlr.M700592-JLR200

Section 2

Therapeutic Aspect Including Iron Metabolism and Heparinase in NAFLD

Chapter 4

Role of the Enzyme Heparanase in the Development of Fatty Liver

Shadi Hamoud

Abstract

Increasing evidence implicates the enzyme Heparanase in the development and progression of liver steatosis and fibrosis, where high heparanase expression was demonstrated. Morever, inhibition of heparanase activity significantly attenuated the development of fatty liver in animal models. Non-alcoholic fatty liver disease is the most common liver disease in the western world, with the natural course of a chronic progressive condition that is expected to worsen with time. Potential complications of the disease are steatohepatitis, liver fibrosis, liver cirrhosis and even liver malignancies, such as hepato-cellular carcinoma. As such, non-alcoholic fatty liver disease is considered a leading etiology for liver transplantation in the western world. No effective treatment for fatty liver is available so far, and seeking effective treatment strategies is of great importance. The aim of this chapter is to shed light on the knowledge regarding the involvement of Heparanase in the development and progression of fatty liver, opening the opportunity for future research of potential therapeutic options for treating this common liver pathology.

Keywords: Heparanase, lipid uptake, liver steatosis, fatty liver, inflammation, extracellular matrix

1. Introduction

The liver is the largest solid organ in the body, and plays important roles in metabolism and processing of nutrients and toxins, with cardinal functions in the gastrointestinal system and the digestion process. The liver is composed of two lobes- right and left, encapsulated by the fibrous Gleason capsule. Cells in the liver are mainly hepatocytes- composing about 60% of the liver cells, sinusoidal endothelial cells (18%), Kupffer cells (KCs 13%), hepatic stellate cells (HSCs, 4–10%), and NK cells (2%) [1–4]. Normally, hepatocytes are arranged in cords surrounding bile canaliculi which drain bile secreted from hepatocytes into bile ducts of the portal triad (**Figure 1**: normal liver).

The extracellular matrix (ECM) is a large network of proteins, glycoseaminoglycans and glycoconjugates and other molecules that surround, support and help to maintain normal structure, function, and integrity of body organs. The ECM helps cells to attach to, and communicate with adjacent cells, and plays important roles in cell growth, cell adhesion, cell movement and migration, and additional cell functions.

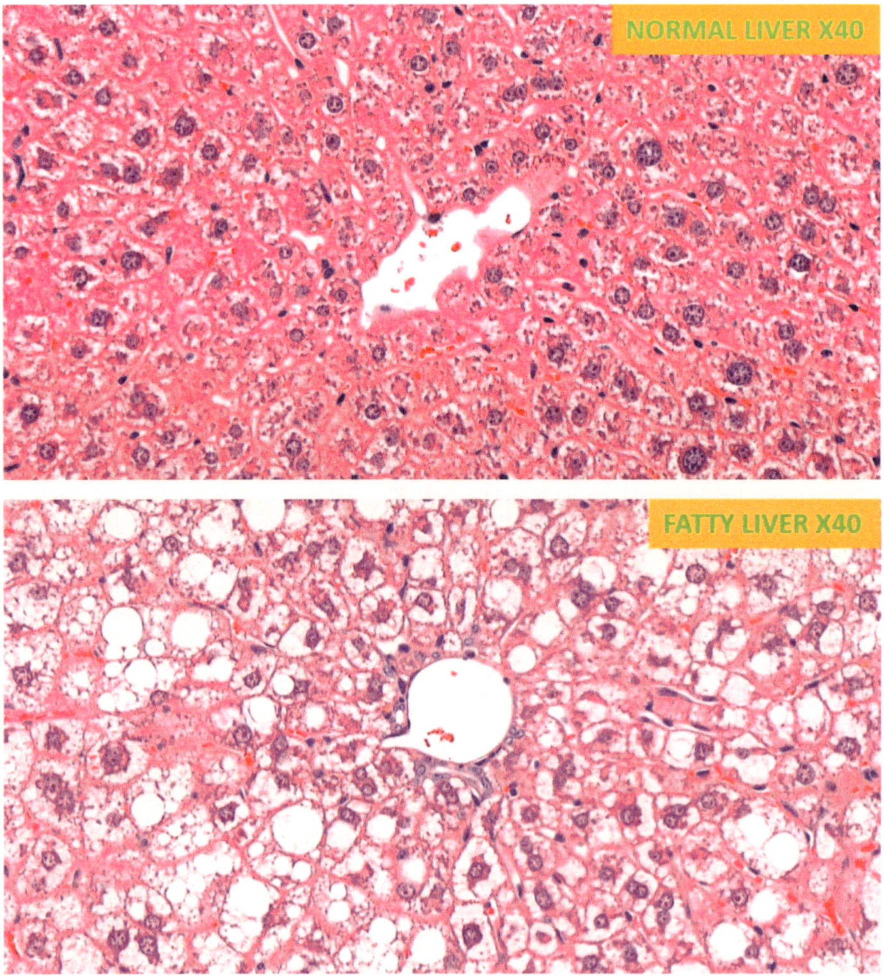

Figure 1.
Structure of normal liver. The liver is composed of two lobes. Hepatocytes are the main cell type in the liver, and are arranged in cords surrounding canaliculi which drain bile into bile ducts to help in digestion of nutrients in the gut. Sections of H&E stained liver slides from normal liver (upper picture) and fatty liver showing intra-cellular vaculations and cell ballooning (lower picture), magnified X40.

Heparan sulfate proteoglycans (HSPG) are the main constituent of the ECM. These macromolecules are composed of glycoseaminoglycan chains covalently bound to a protein core, and are different from each other in their structure and configuration, thus performing different roles in the ECM, which are mainly either adhesive or fibrotic [5]. HSPGs are either embedded in the cell surface or located in the ECM, and play important role in cell-cell and cell-ECM communication and interaction [6–8], thus serve as mediators in both normal biologic and in pathologic processes, like cell differentiation [9, 10], cell adhesion [11], tissue repair [12, 13], tumor formation and spread [5, 10, 14, 15], autoimmune and inflammatory processes [16–18], diabetes mellitus and its complications [19], and vessel wall pathologies- like atherosclerosis [20–22]. Heparanase, an endo-β-D-glucoronidase, is the only enzyme in mammalians that cleaves HS chains in the HSPGs in several specific sites along the polysaccharide chains, thus resulting in modification of structure and function of the HSPGs [21, 23–25]. In its intracellular role, heparanase participates in degradation and turnover of membrane-associated HSPGs [26, 27]. The extracellular enzyme is involved in HSPG degradation by cleavage of the HS chains, resulting in alteration of the basal membrane and ECM structure, and thus affects the pool of HS-bound ligands, which are released into the surrounding environment. All these actions result in remodeling of the ECM network, and enable the diffusion of different cytokines, growth factors, and lipoproteins, which facilitate cell motility and result in angiogenesis, inflammation, coagulation, fibrosis, and stimulation of autophagy and exosome production [28–30].

Non-alcoholic fatty liver disease (NAFLD) is the most common liver disease in the western world, and affects up to 30% of adults [31], with increasing prevalence with age, in line with the global pandemic of obesity and type 2 diabetes mellitus. NAFLD is defined as the intracellular accumulation of fat droplets in the hepatocytes (liver steatosis), as evident by either radiologic or histologic testing, in the absence of alternative etiologies of chronic liver disease or secondary causes of liver steatosis (like the use of various drugs, prolonged alcohol consumption, or inherited or acquired several metabolic pathologies). Isolated NAFLD is characterized by liver steatosis (although could be associated with mild chronic inflammation) in at least 5% of hepatocytes [32]. Natural course of the disease is slow progression to non-alcoholic steatohepatitis (NASH), defined by a pattern of characteristic findings that include liver steatosis, lobular and portal inflammation, and injured liver cells in the form of hepatocyte ballooning. The NAFLD activity score (NAS) is used to assess the degree of hepatic steatosis, lobular inflammation, hepatocellular ballooning, and degree of liver fibrosis [32]. In advanced stages, NAFLD may progress to profound liver fibrosis- as assessed by the METAVIR scoring system, liver cirrhosis, portal hypertension, and end-stage liver diseases with related complications, including liver failure, decompensated liver cirrhosis, and even liver malignancies- like hepatocellular carcinoma (HCC) [33], making NAFLD a leading etiology for liver transplantation in the western world [34–36].

1.1 Normal lipid uptake by the liver cells

Upon food intake, lipid particles in the form of triglycerides (TGs)- the main form of lipids in the food, free cholesterol, and cholesterol ester, undergo emulsification into small lipid particles by bile, and are then hydrolyzed into free fatty acids (FFAs) and monoglycerides by the pancreatic lipase in the small intestine, where these small particles undergo absorption into the blood circulation. After absorption by the intestinal cells, together with phospholipids, cholesterol and proteins, the small lipid particles form chylomicrons that enter the blood from the lymphatic system. The liver is the main organ in the body in which lipid metabolism occurs, and in the liver cells occur processes of lipid digestion, absorption, synthesis, decomposition, and transport.

Most of the lipids in the body are stored in the form of TGs in adipose tissue. FFAs are the main constituents in TGs in body fat, from which they can be dissolved under different circumstances and enter the blood. For being transported in the blood circulation, FFAs bind to albumin, while cholesterol binds to globulin to form lipoproteins, which may contain more TGs in the form of low density lipoprotein cholesterol (LDL-c), or less TGs forming high density lipoprotein cholesterol (HDL-c), and according to the density of the lipoproteins, plasma lipoproteins are divided into four subgroups: chylomicrons, very low density lipoprotein (v-LDL),

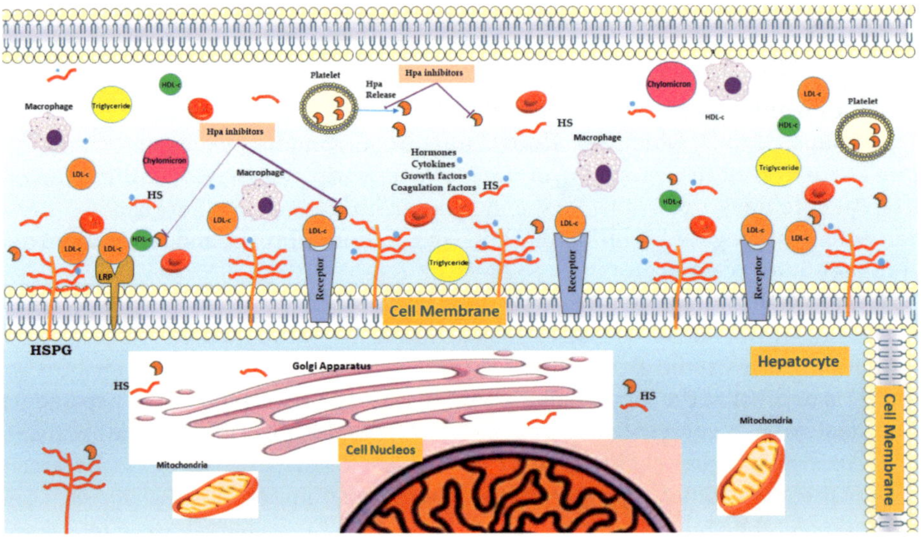

Figure 2.
Schematic presentation of membrane associated structures involved in lipid uptake and metabolism in the liver. Lipid particles ingested in the intestine/formed by lipolysis from fat tissue enter blood circulation, and undergo uptake into hepatocytes utilizing different transmembrane structures, including the low density lipoprotein receptor (LDLR), LDL receptor-related protein (LRP), CD36 and direct endocytosis by heparan sulfate proteoglycanes (HSPGs). Inside the hepatocytes, lipid particles undergo β-oxidation in intra-cellular organelles. HSPGs play rol in lipid uptake and metabolism by hepatocytes. Focus is given to sites where heparanase is active in processing of lipid particles, as well as sites where heparanase inhibition may occur and cause decreased lipid uptake by the hepatocytes. Hpa = Heparanase. LDL-c = low density lipoprotein cholesterol, HDL-c = high density lipoprotein choleterol, HS = heparan sulfate.

LDL, and HDL. Upon binding to lipids, proteins take part in transporting lipids in the plasma, together forming the apolipoproteins (**Figure 2**).

While the main source of fat in the body comes from food ingestion, the body can utilize endogenous fat which is stored mainly in the adipose tissue. In different circumstances, fat in the adipose cells may undergo hydrolyzation into glycerol and FFAs by the enzyme lipase. Upon hydrolysis, glycerol and FFAs are released into the blood and can be used as a source of energy or ingested by the liver cells. HSPGs play important role in lipid uptake by hepatocytes, mainly following removal of the attached lipoprotein particles [37, 38].

1.2 De novo lipogenesis

In addition to fat ingested from diet, hepatocytes can produce fatty acids from the oxidation processes of both glucose and amino acids, and synthesize TGs by acetyl CoA. In fact, hepatocytes can also synthesize endogenous cholesterol by the process of De novo lipogenesis (DNL). Cholesterol biosynthesis in the hepatocytes occurs in the endoplasmic reticulum, and involves more than 30 enzymes, such as aceto-acetyl CoA, and may contribute to the excess accumulation of fat droplets inside the hepatocytes.

1.3 Development of NAFLD

The pathogenetic basis of NAFLD is accumulation in the hepatocytes of lipid droplets which occurs secondary to an imbalance of lipid handling by the liver, when one or more of several mechanisms takes place. Possible mechanisms include excess delivery of free fatty acids (FFAs) to the liver from adipose tissue, increased production of lipids by the liver (De novo lipogenesis), decreased oxidation of fatty acids within the hepatocytes, and impaired export of the TG-rich v-LDL particles. Accumulation of fat droplets in hepatocytes results in cell ballooning and derangement of the normal structure of the liver, and thus induces activation of inflammatory reaction, with activation of HSCs and KCs, which are both involved in the initiation of inflammatory and fibrogenic responses, then leading to the release of proinflammatory cytokines, chemokines, and growth factors, that further augment the inflammatory process and result in activation of HSCs. Of the cytokines released by KCs, tumor growth factor-β (TGF-β), which induces fibrogenesis through activation of HSCs and reactive oxygen substances, leading to accelerated inflammation and progressive liver damage [39], where KCs release also the proinflammatory cytokines TNF-α, IL-6, and IL-β, which also contribute to liver damage. Moreover, following liver insult, both KCs and hepatocytes secrete fibroblast growth factor 2 (FGF-2), which stimulates hepatocyte regeneration and growth, as well as the proliferation and activation of HSCs. Higher levels of FGF-2 result in excess ECM deposition by HSCs, and induce hepatic tissue perturbation and disruption [40, 41]. Upon activation, HSCs transform to α-SMA positive myofibroblasts, which secrete large amounts of ECM proteins causing profound alteration of the extracellular micro-environment. As these processes aim to repair damaged liver tissue, prolonged injury to the liver together with prolonged activation of the repair system result in degradation of the regeneration process, and in late stages may result in uncontrolled fibrogenesis, excess ECM accumulation, and disruption of liver structure [42–45]. Indeed, liver tissue repair is also supported by autophagy, a process by which cells degrade their own components by forming autophagosomes and autolysosomes, and in the liver, autophagy is expected in normal circumstances to result in decreased liver fibrosis [46, 47].

1.4 Development of liver steatosis

While triglycerides are the main lipid component that contributes to the development of fatty liver [48], and account for 60–70% of intrahepatic fat accumulation, also low density lipoprotein (LDL) cholesterol is an important contributor to the development of NAFLD, mainly in cases of high serum LDL levels, where it is known that in subjects with NAFLD, the lipid uptake by the liver is increased, due to enhanced expression on hepatocyte cell surface of the LDL receptor (LDLR), LDL receptor related protein (LRP), and the hepatic fatty acid transporter CD36. In addition, in subjects with high serum levels of lipids, hepatic uptake of lipid particles occurs through direct endocytosis by cell membrane, secondary to increased activity of hepatic lipase and lipoprotein lipase, a process that depends on the activity of HSPGs embedded in the cell wall, in response to augmented insulin resistance that complicates patients with obesity and NAFLD [49, 50].

Following lipid uptake by hepatocytes, lipid particles undergo metabolism and β-oxidation through several intra-cellular metabolic pathways, which include ACAT2, ACAT1, HMGCoA reductase, pPAR-α, pPAR-ɣ, PCSK-9 and DGAT1 [51]. In fact, also De novo lipogenesis contributes to lipid accumulation in the liver of patients with obesity and NAFLD [51, 52]. In this pathway, acetyl CoA and melonyl CoA are converted into fatty acids in the liver, a process that is accelerated in the presence of insulin resistance, which occurs in adjunction with obesity and adiposity [52].

The progression of liver steatosis occurs through several stages. Upon lipid uptake by hepatocytes, fatty acids undergo β-oxidation in mitochondria, peroxisomes, and microsomes, still with existing controversy regarding the rate of lipid oxidation (whether increased or decreased) in patients with NAFLD [51, 53], and accumulation of triglyceride-rich lipoproteins in hepatocytes is increased [51, 54]. Likewise, in patients with NAFLD increased production of small dense LDL-C was demonstrated [55].

The endoplasmic reticulum is the main intra-cellular site for lipid synthesis and protein folding and maturation, and is an important participant in the development of NAFLD, especially in the presence of impaired LDL-Triglyceride assembly, which occurs due to activation of intracellular signaling pathways, in response to higher levels of intracellular lipid particles [56]. Lipotoxicity is more prominent under higher endoplasmic reticulum oxidative stress, that occurs more frequently in obese subjects with NAFLD, apparently due to activation of the unfolded protein response (UPR). One more mechanism that contributes to the development and progression of NAFLD is the accelerated formation of extracellular vesicles, that are nano-sized particles which are over-secreted by hepatocytes in response to higher content of toxic lipid particles, and play critical role in the pathogenesis of NAFLD by acting as mediators of paracrine signaling, causing HSCs activation, angiogenesis and activation of macrophages, all leading to liver inflammation and chemotaxis [57, 58].

1.5 The enzyme heparanase

Heparanase is the only enzyme in mammalians that is responsible for cleavage of HS side chains in the HSPGs. The human heparanase gene (heparanase 1) is located on chromosome 4q21.3 [59]. Also heparanase 2 was demonstrated, sharing 40% similarity with heparanase 1, but does not exert similar activity like heparanase 1 [60]. The enzyme heparanase is synthesized in the endoplasmic reticulum, then processed in the Golgi apparatus to 65 kDa proheparanase, and then released to the extra-cellular space, where it interacts with many membrane molecules, of which are membrane HSPGs like syndecans [61], resulting in endocytosis and localization into the lyzosomes, where it undergoes cleavage to its two active forms- 50 and 6 kDa. It was proven that the active enzyme has several final destinations in the cell: it could undergo anchorage on the surface of exosomes, included in autophagosomes, translocated into cell nucleus, or even be secreted to the ECM [62]. The enzyme expresses both enzymatic and non-enzymatic activities, inside the cell and in the ECM. In its enzymatic intracellular role, activity of heparanase is mainly degradation and turnover of membrane-associated HSPGs. The extracellular enzymatic activity is mainly degradation of transmembrane and ECM located HSPGs, leading both to alterations in structure and function of HSPGs in the ECM, and resulting in attenuation of HS-bound ligands and proteins which are released into the surrounding environment, causing diffusion of cytokines, growth factors, and lipoproteins, and facilitating cell motility, angiogenesis, inflammation, coagulation, and stimulating autophagic and exosome production [63–67].

Non-enzymatic activity of heparanase has been demonstrated, although the receptors that could mediate this activity have not been identified so far. Of the non-enzymatic activities of the enzyme, one can mention that the heparanase proenzyme (65 kDa) was demonstrated to induce signaling cascade towards phosphorylation of several proteins, including those involved in intracellular signaling pathways, such as Akt, ERK, p38, and Src [68]. Of the resultant effects of this activity were noted endothelial cell migration and invasion, which are enhanced by the proheparanase-Akt phosphorylation and activation of PI3K [69]. Moreover, latent heparanase was implicated in induction of tumorogenesis, such as the development of glioma, lymphoma, and T-cell adhesion, apparently due to activation of Akt, PyK2 and ERK, and Akt/PKB phosphorylation [70].

2. Heparanase in liver pathologies

2.1 Heparanase in viral hepatitis

As viruses utilize membrane structure for invading cells, HSPGs are involved in the process of cell infection and inclusion of viruses into host cells [71]. In their study, Gallard et al. demonstrated that hepatitis C virus (HCV) propagation resulted in significant heparanase induction in hepatocytes, while downregulation of heparanase resulted in significant attenuation of HCV infection, suggesting an important role of heparanase in HCV life cycle. Heparanase action was apparently secondary to enhancement of CD63 synthesis and exosomic secretion [72].

2.2 Heparanase in liver fibrosis

In their book chapter, Mazola et al. suggest that the interplay between heparanase and components of the immune and the inflammatory responses activate recruitment, proliferation, and activation of myofibroblasts, the main cell types responsible for deposition of fibrous proteins in the ECM [73]. In a study on mice with chronic Ccl4-mediated chronic induction of liver fibrosis, increased heparanase expression was demonstrated, which was mainly co-localized with macrophages in necro-inflammatory areas, where it seems that heparanase plays a key role in the macrophage-mediated activation of HSCs [74]. Further studies supported additional evidence for the involvement of heparanase in fibrotic processes in different body organs, including liver fibrosis [75].

2.3 Heparanase in malignant diseases of the liver

The expression of heparanase in malignant diseases has been extensively studied, including the effects of several heparanase inhibitors that were evaluated in several malignant diseases. In one study, it was shown that heparanase-1 degrades the HS chains on cells of hepatocellular carcinoma (HCC), a process that resulted in the secretion of vascular endothelial growth factor C (VEGF-C) into the medium of HCC cells, while VEGF-C was shown to promote lymphatic endothelial cell growth leading to facilitating lymphatic metastasis [76]. Chen et al. showed elevated expression of heparanase mRNA and protein in HCC cells, where it accelerates cell adhesion in HCC metastasis, an effect that was significantly attenuated following silencing of the enzyme [77]. In the study of Liu et al., the authors showed that inhibiting heparanase activity by the inhibitor PI-88 exerted favorable effects in patients with HCC. Heparanase inhibition resulted in significant delay in the onset of recurrence of HCC, and provided significant survival benefit for up to three years of follow up [78].

2.4 Heparanase inhibition and liver steatosis

In our former studies, we investigated the effect of heparanase inhibition on hemodynamic, metabolic and histopathologic parameters of body systems in mice, mainly aortic atherosclerosis and fatty liver.

In apolipoprotein E deficient (E0) mice, inhibition of heparanase activity by two inhibitors- PG545 (PIXATIMOD), a HS mimetic with proved inhibitory effect on heparanase, caused significant reduction of serum glucose levels, blood pressure and oxidative stress in serum [79]. In another project, we have shown that the same heparanase inhibitor, used in E0 mice placed on high fat diet, significantly attenuated the development of atherosclerotic lesions in representing sections taken from the aortic arch, along significant reduction of the aortic wall thickness compared to control mice. In addition, we demonstrated in the same study that in comparison to placebo, treatment with PG545 significantly reduced blood pressure and serum levels of TC, TGs, and LDL-C, besides significant reduction of oxidative stress in serum, all of which are considered independent risk factors for the development and progression of atherosclerosis [80].

Recently, we studied the effect of two different heparanase inhibitors on the development of liver steatosis in two kinds of mice. In this study, both E0 mice and C57 Balb-c mice were placed on either chow diet or high fat diet, and treated with either PG545, SST0001- a 100% N-acetylated and glycol split non-anticoagulant heparin which exerts potent anti heparanase activity, or placebo injection (normal saline). Both heparanase inhibitors significantly attenuated the development of liver steatosis. In accordance with our former studies, also in this study serum analyses revealed significant reduction in serum levels of TC and TGs, besides lowering the mRNA expression of key factors involved lipid metabolism, including lipid uptake by the liver, lipolysis, lipogenesis, and beta-oxidation in the liver cells. These beneficial effects seem to heparanase-dependent, as inhibition of heparanase resulted in the favorable effect of attenuating the development of fatty liver [81].

3. Conclusions/concluding remarks

Non-alcoholic fatty liver disease is the most common liver disease in the western world. Yet, the mechanisms underlying the pathogenesis of this formidable is largely vague, thus lacks effective treatment so far. HSPGs are the main constituent of the extracellular matrix, and play important roles in liver pathologies, through cell-cell and cell-ECM interactions, besides their role in uptake and processing of lipid particles by the liver cells. Heparanase is the enzyme that degrades heparan sulfate side chains in HSPGs, involves in remodeling of structure and alter the function of the HSPG macromolecules. Heparanase inhibition was proved to exert favorable results in different pathologies, including malignant diseases, complications of diabetes mellitus, kidney pathologies, inflammatory processes, and vessel wall pathologies like atherosclerosis. Recently we have demonstrated remarkable attenuation in the development of fatty liver in animal models with the use of two different heparanase inhibitors, an additional evidence for the involvement of heparanase in the development of fatty liver, putting heparanase inhibition as a reliable target for future research concerning the development of possible effective treatment for NAFLD. It could be wise to impliment heparanase inhibition as a part of treatment approach for preventing and treating NAFLD, along with restriction of lipid uptake, preventing weight gain and weight, and optimal control of additional conditions that contribute to the development of NAFLD, such insulin resistance and diabetes mellitus.

Acknowledgements

Thanks for Professor Z. Abassi from the Department of Physiology and Biophysics, the Bruce Rappaport Faculty of Medicine, Technion, Haifa, Israel, for his valuable assistance.

Conflict of interest

No conflict of interest to be declared.

Author details

Shadi Hamoud
Rambam Health Care Campus and Rappaport Faculty of Medicine, Technion, Israel Institute of Technology, Department of Internal Medicine E, Haifa, Israel

*Address all correspondence to: s_hamoud@rmc.gov.il

References

[1] Sasse D, Spornitz UM, Maly IP. Liver architecture. Enzyme. 1992;**46**:8-32 [PubMed] [Google Scholar]

[2] Knook DL, Sleyster EC. Isolated parenchymal, Kupffer and endothelial rat liver cells characterized by their lysosomal enzyme content. Biochemical and Biophysical Research Communications. 1980;**96**:250-257 [PubMed] [Google Scholar]

[3] Blouin A, Bolender RP, Weibel ER. Distribution of organelles and membranes between hepatocytes and nonhepatocytes in the rat liver parenchyma. A stereological study. The Journal of Cell Biology. 1977;**72**:441-455 [PMC free article] [PubMed] [Google Scholar]

[4] Weibel ER, Stäubli W, Gnägi HR, Hess FA. Correlated morphometric and biochemical studies on the liver cell. I. Morphometric model, stereologic methods, and normal morphometric data for rat liver. The Journal of Cell Biology. 1969;**42**:68-91 [PMC free article] [PubMed] [Google Scholar]

[5] Vlodavsky I, Blich M, Li JP, Sanderson RD, Ilan N. Involvement of heparanase in atherosclerosis and other vessel wall pathologies. Matrix Biology. 2013;**32**(5):241e251

[6] Bernfield M, Gotte M, Park PW, Reizes O, Fitzgerald ML, Lincecum J, et al. Functions of cell surface heparan sulfate proteoglycans. Annual Review of Biochemistry. 1999;**68**:729e777

[7] Ilan N, Elkin M, Vlodavsky I. Regulation, function and clinical significance of heparanase in cancer metastasis and angiogenesis. The International Journal of Biochemistry & Cell Biology. 2006;**38**(12):2018e2039

[8] Sasisekharan R, Shriver Z, Venkataraman G, Narayanasami U. Roles of heparan-sulphate glycosaminoglycans in cancer. Nature Reviews Cancer. 2002;**2**(7):521e528

[9] Vlodavsky I, Friedmann I. Molecular properties and involvement of heparanase in cancer metastasis and angiogenesis. The Journal of Clinical Investigation. 2001;**108**(3):341-347

[10] Parish CR, Freeman C, Hulett MD. Heparanase: A key enzyme involved in cell invasion, Biochimica et Biophysica Acta (BBA) – Reviews on. Cancer. 2001;**1471**(3):M99-M108

[11] Zetser A, Bashenko Y, Edovitsky E, Levy-Adam F, Vlodavsky I, Ilan N. Heparanase induces vascular endothelial growth factor expression: Correlation with p38 phosphorylation levels and Src activation. Cancer Research. 2006;**66**(3):1455-1463

[12] Barash U, Cohen-Kaplan V, Dowek I, Sanderson RD, Ilan N, Vlodavsky I. Proteoglycans in health and disease: New concepts for heparanase function in tumor progression and metastasis. FEBS Journal. 2010;**277**(19):3890-3903

[13] Sandwall E, O'Callaghan P, Zhang X, Lindahl U, Lannfelt L, Li J. Heparan sulfate mediates amyloid-beta internalization and cytotoxicity. Glycobiology. 2010;**20**(5):533-541

[14] Lygizos MI, Yang Y, Altmann CJ, Okamura K, Andres Hernando A, Perez MJ, et al. Heparanase mediates renal dysfunction during early sepsis in mice. Physiological Reports. 2013;**1**(6): e00153. DOI: 10.1002/phy2.153

[15] Goldberg R, Rubinstein AM, Gil N, Hermano E, Li JP, Van der Vlag J, et al. Role of heparanase-driven inflammatory cascade in pathogenesis of diabetic nephropathy. Diabetes. 2014;**63**(12):4302-4313

[16] Assady S, Alter J, Axelman E, Zohar Y, Sabo E, Litvak M, et al. Nephroprotective effect of heparanase in experimental nephrotic syndrome. PLoS One. 2015;**10**(3):e0119610

[17] Szymczak M, Kuzniar J, Klinger M. The role of heparanase in diseases of the glomeruli. Archivum Immunologiae et Therapiae Experimentalis. 2010;**58**(1):45-56

[18] Van Den Hoven MJ, Rops AL, Vlodavsky I, Levidiotis V, Berden JH, Van Der Vlag J. Heparanase in glomerular diseases. Kidney International. 2007;**72**(5):543-548

[19] Levidiotis V, Freeman C, Tikellis C, Cooper ME, Power DA. Heparanase is involved in the pathogenesis of proteinuria as a result of glomerulonephritis. Journal of the American Society of Nephrology. 2004;**15**(1):68-78

[20] Kramer A, Van Den Hoven M, Rops A, Wijnhoven T, van den Heuvel L, Lensen J, et al. Induction of glomerular heparanase expression in rats with adriamycin nephropathy is regulated by reactive oxygen species and the renin-angiotensin system. Journal of the American Society of Nephrology. 2006;**17**(9):2513-2520

[21] Van den Hoven MJ, Waanders F, Rops AL, Kramer AB, van Goor H, Berden JH, et al. Regulation of glomerular heparanase expression by aldosterone, angiotensin II and reactive oxygen species. Nephrology Dialysis Transplantation. 2009;**24**(9):2637-2645

[22] Levidiotis V, Freeman C, Tikellis C, Cooper ME, Power DA. Heparanase inhibition reduces proteinuria in a model of accelerated anti-glomerular basement membrane antibody disease. Nephrology. 2005;**10**(2):167-173

[23] Tao YH, Wang Z, Zhou YR. Expression of heparanase in kidney of rats with respiratory syncytial virus nephropathy and its relationship with proteinurina. Sichuan Da Xue Xue Bao. Yi Xue Ban. 2014;**45**(2):212-215

[24] Levidiotis V, Kanellis J, Ierino FL, Power DA. Increased expression of heparanase in puromycin aminonucleoside nephrosis. Kidney International. 2001;**60**(4):1287-1296

[25] Masola V, Zaza G, Gambaro G, Onisto M, Bellin G, Vischini G, et al. Heparanase: A potential new factor involved in the renal epithelial mesenchymal transition (EMT) induced by ischemia/reperfusion (I/R) injury. PLoS One. 2016;**11**(7):e0160074

[26] Vreys V, David G. Mammalian heparanase: What is the message? Journal of Cellular and Molecular Medicine. 2007;**11**:427, [CrossRef] [PubMed]-452

[27] Secchi MF, Masola V, Zaza G, Lupo A, Gambaro G, Onisto M. Recent data concerning heparanase: Focus on fibrosis, inflammation and cancer. Biomolecular Concepts. 2015;**6**:415-421 [CrossRef]

[28] Barbouri D, Afratis N, Gialeli C, Vynios DH, Theocharis AD, Karamanos NK. Syndecans as modulators and potential pharmacological targets in cancer progression. Frontiers in Oncology. 2014;**4**:4. DOI: 10.3389/fonc.2014.00004

[29] Gomes AM, Stelling MP, Pavo MSG. Heparan sulfate and heparanase as

modulators of breast cancer progression. BioMed Research International. 2013;**2013**:852093. DOI: 10.1155/2013/852093

[30] Ramani V.C, Purushothaman A, Stewart M.D, Thompson C.A, Vlodavsky I, Au J.L-S, Sanderson R.D. The heparanase/syndecan-1 axis in cancer: Mechanisms and therapies. The FEBS Journal, 2013, 280, 2294-2306

[31] Younossi ZM, Koenig AB, Abdelatif D, Fazel Y, Henry L, Wymer M. Global epidemiology of nonalcoholic fatty liver disease- meta-analytic assessment of prevalence, incidence, and outcomes. Hepatology. 2016;**64**:73-84 [CrossRef]

[32] Kleiner DE, Brunt EM, Van Natta M, Behling C, Contos MJ, Cummings OW, et al. Nonalcoholic steatohepatitis clinical research network. Design and validation of a histological scoring system for nonalcoholic fatty liver disease. Hepatology. 2005;**41**(6):1313-1321. DOI: 10.1002/hep.20701

[33] Chalasani N, Younossi Z, Lavine JE, Diehl AM, Brunt EM, Cusi K, et al. The diagnosis and management of non-alcoholic fatty liver disease: Practice guideline by the American Gastroenterological Association, American Association for the Study of Liver Diseases, and American College of Gastroenterology. Gastroenterology. 2012;**142**(7):1592-1609 [PubMed: 22656328]

[34] Dixon LJ, Barnes M, Tang H, Pritchard MT, Nagy LE. Kupffer cells in the liver. Comprehensive Physiology. 2013;**3**:785, [CrossRef] [PubMed]-797

[35] Puche JE, Saiman Y, Friedman SL. Hepatic stellate cells and liver fibrosis. Comprehensive Physiology. 2013;**3**:1473, [CrossRef] [PubMed]-1492

[36] Wong RJ, Singal AK. Trends in liver disease etiology among adults awaiting liver transplantation in the United States, 2014-2019. JAMA Network Open. 2020;**3**:e1920294 [CrossRef] [PubMed]

[37] Nguyen P, Leray V, Diez M, Serisier S, Le Bloc'h J, Siliart B, et al. Liver lipid metabolism. Journal of Animal Physiology & Animal Nutrition. 2010;**92**(3):272-283

[38] Sunami Y, Rebelo A, Kleeff J. Lipid metabolism and lipid droplets in pancreatic cancer and stellate cells. Cancers. 2018;**10**(1):3

[39] Sato K, Hall C, Glaser S, Francis H, Meng F, Alpini G. Pathogenesis of Kupffer cells in Cholestatic liver injury. The American Journal of Pathology. 2016;**186**:2238-2247 [CrossRef]

[40] Schumacher J.D, Guo G.L. Regulation of hepatic stellate cells and Fibrogenesis by fibroblast growth factors. BioMed Research International 2016, 2016, 8323747. [CrossRef] [PubMed]

[41] Yu C, Wang F, Jin C, Huang X, Miller DL, Basilico C, et al. Role of fibroblast growth factor type 1 and 2 in carbon tetrachloride-induced hepatic injury and fibrogenesis. The American Journal of Pathology. 2003;**163**:1653-1662 [CrossRef]

[42] Pellicoro A, Ramachandran P, Iredale JP, Fallowfield JA. Liver fibrosis and repair: Immune regulation of wound healing in a solid organ. Nature Reviews. Immunology. 2014;**14**:181, [CrossRef] [PubMed]-194

[43] Wong RJ, Aguilar M, Cheung R, Perumpail RB, Harrison SA, Younossi ZM, et al. Nonalcoholic steatohepatitis is the second leading etiology of liver disease among adults awaiting liver

transplantation in the United States. Gastroenterology. 2015;**148**:547-555 [CrossRef]

[44] Charlton MR, Burns JM, Pedersen RA, Watt KD, Heimbach JK, Dierkhising RA. Frequency and outcomes of liver transplantation for nonalcoholic steatohepatitis in the United States. Gastroenterology. 2011;**141**:1249, [CrossRef] [PubMed]-1253

[45] Welzel TM, Graubard BI, Quraishi S, Zeuzem S, Davila JA, El-Serag HB, et al. Population-attributable fractions of risk factors for hepatocellular carcinoma in the United States. The American Journal of Gastroenterology. 2013;**108**:1314, [CrossRef] [PubMed]-1321

[46] Thoen LF, Guimaraes EL, Dolle L, Mannaerts I, Najimi M, Sokal E, van Grunsven LA. A role for autophagy during hepatic stellate cell activation. Journal of Hepatology. 2011;**55**:1353-1360. [CrossRef] [PubMed]

[47] Li Y, Chen Y, Huang H, Shi M, Yang W, Kuang J, et al. Autophagy mediated by endoplasmic reticulum stress enhances the caffeine-induced apoptosis of hepatic stellate cells. International Journal of Molecular Medicine. 2017;**377**:2063-2072. [PubMed]-1414

[48] Diehl AM, Day C. Cause, Pathogenesis, and treatment of nonalcoholic steatohepatitis. The New England Journal of Medicine 2017, 377, 2063-2072. [CrossRef] [PubMed]

[49] Geisler CE, Renquist BJ. Hepatic lipid accumulation: Cause and consequence of dysregulated glucoregulatory hormones. The Journal of Endocrinology. 2017;**234**(1):R1-R21

[50] Miksztowicz V, Lucero D, Zago V, Cacciagiú L, Lopez G, Gonzalez Ballerga E, et al. Hepatic lipase activity is increased in non-alcoholic fatty liver disease beyond insulin resistance. Diabetes/Metabolism Research and Reviews. 2012;**28**(6):535-541

[51] Fabbrini E, Tiemann Luecking C, Love-Gregory L, Okunade AL, Yoshino M, Fraterrigo G, et al. Physiological mechanisms of weight gaininduced steatosis in people with obesity. Gastroenterology. 2016;**150**(1):79-81

[52] Donnelly KL, Smith CI, Schwarzenberg SJ, Jessurun J, Boldt MD, Parks EJ. Sources of fatty acids stored in liver and secreted via lipoproteins in patients with nonalcoholic fatty liver disease. Journal of Clinical Investigation. 2005;**115**(5):1343-1351

[53] Afolabi PR, Scorletti E, Smith DE, Almehmadi AA, Calder PC, Byrne CD. The characterisation of hepatic mitochondrial function in patients with non-alcoholic fatty liver disease (NAFLD) using the (13) C-ketoisocaproate breath test. Journal of Breath Research. 2018;**12**(4):046002

[54] Fabbrini E, Mohammed BS, Magkos F, Korenblat KM, Patterson BW, Klein S. Alterations in adipose tissue and hepatic lipid kinetics in obese men and women with nonalcoholic fatty liver disease. Gastroenterology. 2008;**134**(2):424-431

[55] Fon Tacer K, Rozman D. Nonalcoholic fatty liver disease: Focus on lipoprotein and lipid deregulation. 2011:783976:14. DOI: 10.1155/2011/783976

[56] Lebeaupin C, Vallée D, Hazari Y, Hetz C, Chevet E, Bailly-Maitre B. Endoplasmic reticulum stress signalling and the pathogenesis of non-alcoholic fatty liver disease. Journal of Hepatology. 2018;**69**(4):927-947

[57] Hernández A, Arab JP, Reyes D, Lapitz A, Moshage H, Bañales JM, et al. Extracellular vesicles in NAFLD/ALD: From pathobiology to therapy. Cell. 2020;**9**(4):817. DOI: 10.3390/cells9040817

[58] Hirsova P, Ibrahim SH, Krishnan A, Verma VK, Bronk SF, Werneburg NW, et al. Lipid-induced signaling causes release of inflammatory extracellular vesicles from hepatocytes. Gastroenterology. 2016;**150**(4):956-967

[59] Lee YS, Kim SY, Ko E, Lee JH, Yi HS, Yoo YJ, et al. Exosomes derived from palmitic acid-treated hepatocytes induce fibrotic activation of hepatic stellate cells. Scientific Reports. 2017;7(1):3710

[60] Rivara S, Milazzo FM, Giannini G. Heparanase: A rainbow pharmacological target associated to multiple pathologies including rare diseases. Future. Medicinal Chemistry. 2016;**8**:647, [CrossRef] [PubMed]-680

[61] Vlodavsky I, Gross-Cohen M, Weissmann M, Ilan N, Sanderson RD. Opposing functions of Heparanase-1 and Heparanase-2 in cancer progression. Trends in Biochemical Sciences. 2018;**43**:18. [CrossRef] [PubMed]-31

[62] Gong F, Jemth P, Escobar Galvis ML, Vlodavsky I, Horner A, Lindahl U, et al. Processing of macromolecular heparin by heparanase. The Journal of Biological Chemistry. 2003;**278**:35152. [CrossRef] [PubMed]-35158

[63] Vlodavsky I, Singh P, Boyango I, Gutter-Kapon L, Elkin M, Sanderson RD, et al. Heparanase: From basic research to therapeutic applications in cancer and inflammation. Drug Resistance Updates. 2016;**29**:54-75

[64] Sanderson RD, Elkin M, Rapraeger AC, Ilan N, Vlodavsky I. Heparanase regulation of cancer, autophagy and inflammation: New mechanisms and targets for therapy. The FEBS Journal. 2017;**284**:42-55. [CrossRef] [PubMed]

[65] Meirovitz A, Goldberg R, Binder A, Rubinstein AM, Hermano E, Elkin M. Heparanase in inflammation and inflammation-associated cancer. The FEBS Journal. 2013;**280**:2307. [CrossRef] [PubMed]-2319

[66] Sanderson RD, Bandari SK, Vlodavsky I. Proteases and glycosidases on the surface of exosomes: Newly discovered mechanisms for extracellular remodeling. Matrix Biology. 2019;**75-76**: 160-169. ISSN 0945-053X. DOI: 10.1016/j.matbio.2017.10.007

[67] Jin H, Zhou S. The functions of heparanase in human diseases. Mini Reviews in Medicinal Chemistry. 2017;**17**:541-548

[68] Fux L, Ilan N, Sanderson RD, Vlodavsky I. Heparanase: Busy at the cell surface. Trends in Biochemical Sciences. 2009;**34**:511. [CrossRef] [PubMed]-519

[69] Gingis-Velitski S, Zetser A, Flugelman MY, Vlodavsky I, Ilan N. Heparanase induces endothelial cell migration via protein kinase B/Akt activation. The Journal of Biological Chemistry. 2004;**279**:23536-23541. [CrossRef] [PubMed])

[70] Ben-Zaken O, Gingis-Velitski S, Vlodavsky I, Ilan N. Heparanase induces Akt phosphorylation via a lipid raft receptor. Biochemical and Biophysical Research Communications. 2007;**361**:829-834

[71] Cagno V, Tseligka E, Jones ST, Tapparel C. Heparan sulfate proteoglycans and viral attachment: True receptors or adaptation bias? Viruses. 2019;**11**:596. DOI: 10.3390/v11070596

[72] Gallard C, Lebsir N, Khursheed H, Reungoat E, Plissonnier ML, Bré J, et al. Heparanase-1 is upregulated by hepatitis C virus and favors its replication. Journal of Hepatology. 2022;77(1):29-41. DOI: 10.1016/j.jhep.2022.01.008 Epub 2022 Jan 25

[73] Masola V, Gambaro G, Onisto M. Impact of Heparanse on organ fibrosis. Advances in Experimental Medicine and Biology. 2020;**1221**:669-684. DOI: 10.1007/978-3-030-34521-1_27

[74] Secchi MF, Crescenzi M, Masola V, Russo FP, Floreani A, Onisto M. Heparanase and macrophage interplay in the onset of liver fibrosis. Scientific Reports. 2017;7(1):14956. DOI: 10.1038/s41598-017-14946-0

[75] Lv Q, Zeng J, He L. The advancements of heparanase in fibrosis. International Journal of Molecular Epidemiology and Genetics. 2016;7(4):137-140

[76] Yu S, Lv H, Zhang H, Jiang Y, Hong Y, Xia R, et al. Heparanase-1-induced shedding of heparan sulfate from syndecan-1 in hepatocarcinoma cell facilitates lymphatic endothelial cell proliferation via VEGF-C/ERK pathway. Biochemical and Biophysical Research Communications. 2017;**485**(2):432-439. DOI: 10.1016/j.bbrc.2017.02.060 Epub 2017 Feb 13

[77] Peng C, Ren P, Zhou Q, Sun Q, Zhao X, Cong B. Heparanase antisense suppression of A-549 lung carcinoma invasion. Asian Pacific Journal of Cancer Prevention. 2011;**12**(12):3371-3374

[78] Liu CJ, Chang J, Lee PH, Lin DY, Wu CC, Jeng LB, et al. Adjuvant heparanase inhibitor PI-88 therapy for hepatocellular carcinoma recurrence. World Journal of Gastroenterology. 2014;**20**(32):11384-11393. DOI: 10.3748/wjg. v20. i32.11384

[79] Hamoud S, Shekh-Muhammad R, Abu-Saleh N, Hassan A, Zohar Y, Hayek T. Heparanase inhibition reduces glucose levels, blood pressure, and oxidative stress in apolipoprotein E knockout mice. BioMed Research International. 2017. Article ID 7357495. DOI: 10.1155/2017/7357495

[80] Muhammad RS, Abu-Saleh N, Kinaneh S, Agbaria M, Sabo E, Grajeda-Iglesias C, et al. Heparanase inhibition attenuates atherosclerosis progression and liver steatosis in E0 mice. Atherosclerosis. 2018;**276**:155e162

[81] Kinaneh S, Hijaze W, Mansour-Wattad L, Hammoud R, Zaidani H, Kabala A, et al. Heparanase inhibition prevents liver steatosis in E0 mice. Journal of Clinical Medicine. 2022;**11**:1672. DOI: 10.3390/jcm11061672), 10.3390/jcm11061672)

Chapter 5

Regulation of Iron Metabolism in NAFLD/NASH

Yuki Hamada and Eiichi Hirano

Abstract

The disturbance of iron metabolism is one of the characteristic features of NAFLD/NASH, and complicated Type2DM, however, as for the mechanisms of the iron deposition observed in the liver of NAFLD/NASH, as well as the correlation between iron metabolism and insulin resistance, the precise pathophysiology and dynamics are still uncertain. In addition, numerous factors might be involved in the pathogenesis of NAFLD/NASH and wide-ranged analysis, as well as multi-targeted treatment, should be considered and challenged for the improvement of the prognosis of NAFLD/NASH. In many NAFLD/NASH cases, a remarkable decline of serum ferritin, as well as the improvement of T2DM, were observed after treatment with Laennec (placenta-derived drug) in accordance with the improvement of the liver dysfunction and histopathological amelioration in the liver. In recent years, it was shown that hepcidin, the principal regulator of iron metabolism exists in human placenta in high concentrations. Then, we examined whether Laennec can restore the pathological background by regulating iron and glucose metabolism in NAFLD/NASH by the action of a "hepcidin inducer".

Keywords: non-alcoholic fatty liver disease (NAFLD), non-alcoholic steatohepatitis (NASH), iron metabolism, hepcidin, placenta extract

1. Introduction

Non-alcoholic fatty liver disease (NAFLD), regarded as the 'hepatic manifestation of the metabolic syndrome', is now estimated to affect one billion individuals worldwide [1]. The definition of NAFLD is very simple such as the presence of at least 5% hepatic steatosis but excluding secondary hepatic fat accumulation of general causes, such as congenital hepatic disorders, chronic viral hepatitis, autoimmune hepatitis, excessive alcohol consumption, or long-term use of steatosis-inducing medications [2].

NASH is characterised by the development of histopathological changes in the liver that are nearly identical to those induced by excessive alcohol intake, but in the absence of alcohol abuse, the presence of macrovesicular steatosis and mixed inflammatory infiltrate associated with focal hepatocyte ballooning degeneration and varying amounts of Mallory's hyaline and glycogenated nuclei. However, liver biopsy still remains the "gold standard" for making a definitive diagnosis.

NASH is capable of progressing to cirrhosis and liver failure at the end of clinical course [3, 4]. Actually, NASH is forecasted to become the principal cause of advanced liver disease in developed countries [5] and the high-ranking indication for liver transplantation [4]. NAFLD has also been gradually acknowledged as an independent risk factor for the development of cardiovascular disease, type 2 diabetes mellitus (T2DM) and hepatocellular carcinoma [6, 7]. The factors that predispose patients to the development of steatohepatitis and fibrosis in NAFLD are not well elucidated, and effective treatment strategies are still lacking [8].

Day and James [9] initially proposed a 'two-hit' model to explain the progression of NAFLD. The 'first hit' constitutes the deposition of triglycerides in the cytoplasm of the hepatocytes. The disease does not progress unless additional cellular events occur (the 'second hit'), which can include oxidative stress, especially that arises from inflammatory cytokines, mitochondrial stress and insulin resistance. Autophagy may also play a notable role in the pathogenesis of NASH.

A new prospect explaining the pathogenesis of NASH was reported by Tilg and Moschen, called the 'multi-parallel hit' hypothesis recently [10]. This hypothesis, based on reports that cytokine-mediated stress and endoplasmic reticulum stress can induce steatosis as well as necroinflammation, suggests that multiple hits take a step together in the development of NASH. The progression of steatosis should, therefore, be regarded as a part of the liver's early 'adaptive' and 'purposive' response to some types of stress rather than as the first hit in the disease development. The close correlation between insulin resistance and iron level has been speculated and examined by many researchers. Even if secondary iron accumulation increases insulin resistance or vice versa, it remains still unclear. Oxidative stress may be the elusive 'second' hit of possibly multiple steps in the progression of steatosis to fibrosing steatohepatitis [11]. This type of response might be originated from and been modified by the activation of hepatic stellate cells (HSCs) [12].

2. Relationship between NASH/NAFLD and iron metabolism

Iron is among the essential trace elements for the existence of all living organisms. It is required for numerous metabolic routines, including energy production, DNA synthesis, oxygen transport and innate immunity, also in the expression of other enzymes involved in the oxidation or reduction of biological substrates and in the activation of iron-containing enzymes, such as the cytochrome system in the mitochondria [13]. Because there is no known physiological mechanism for appropriately and efficiently eliminating the 'too much incorporated' iron, even in severe iron-overloaded conditions, a crucial element in maintaining systemic iron homeostasis is effective and harmonised correspondence among cells that use iron (mainly erythroid precursors), absorb iron from the diet (duodenal enterocytes) and store iron (hepatocytes and tissue macrophages). Therefore, when the iron intake exceeds the cellular provisions and storage capabilities are overflowed, iron toxicity due to overloading may easily develop [14]. Thus, iron balance is maintained through steady and urbane regulatory mechanisms.

Recent studies have established the importance of hepcidin in iron homeostasis as a negative regulator of iron release into the bloodstream by duodenal enterocytes and reticuloendothelial macrophages [15]. Excess iron in the liver promotes steatohepatitis, liver fibrosis, cirrhosis and hepatocellular carcinoma [16]. The discovery of hepcidin and the elucidation of its role in iron metabolism made it possible to develop novel therapies for hemochromatosis, anaemia of inflammation and other iron-related disorders such as NAFLD/NASH [17]. Hepcidin has a distinct and essential role in controlling the dietary absorption of iron, its storage and its release into the bloodstream. Hepcidin concentrations are strictly controlled, and their pathologic dysregulation leads to numerous human iron-related disorders such as NAFLD/NASH. Our understanding of hepcidin regulation has rapidly increased; however, numerous questions related to hepcidin pathobiology still need to be clarified and addressed [18].

Iron is stringently and elegantly regulated by a mechanism similar to that for glucose control [19]. Like glucose and insulin, the serum iron levels are regulated by a hepatic peptide hormone, hepcidin. Elevated iron levels arouse hepcidin synthesis, which decreases the levels of the iron-exporter ferroportin in macrophages and intestinal cells and reduces serum iron levels, similar to how insulin controls excessive glucose levels [19, 20].

The spectrum of NAFLD ranges from simple steatosis to NASH [21]. Iron is regarded as a putative element that interacts with oxygen radicals, and NASH is associated with high rates of hyperferritinemia together with increased hepatic iron stores [22]. The role of hepatic iron in the progression and pathogenesis of NASH remains unclear and controversial.

It stands to reason that iron is one of the most copious metals on the earth with the potential of high toxicity against living cells. Highly active cells need iron for maintaining their metabolic activity because iron allows optimal and preferable electron transfer, assisting biochemical reactions between different atoms and molecules. The toxicity of iron originated from induction of reactive oxygen species (ROS), which at high levels leads to cellular damage [23, 24]. Progress in understanding the involvement of hepcidin in normal physiology and disease conditions [25], coupled with advances in quantification, make it an increasingly attractive candidate biomarker for assessing iron status and guiding iron intervention strategies [26]. Evidence suggests that a modest degree of iron overload is associated with more advanced liver injury in NAFLD, although the mechanisms by which this might occur remain unclear and vague [27, 28].

Recently, however, it has become increasingly evident that iron in the adipose tissue plays an important role in the pathogenesis of insulin resistance and, therefore, possibly NAFLD [29, 30].

Excessive iron is also a potent cause of cellular injury from oxidative stress due to the generation of reactive oxygen species by the Fenton reaction [31]. Under usual conditions, intracellular protection from iron-induced oxidative stress is facilitated by the sequestration of iron within ferritin [32]. Dysfunctional adipose tissue produces adipokines that promote the development of insulin resistance [29]. The liver, skeletal muscle and adipose tissue are the key sites of insulin action and resistance [33]. In the adipose tissue itself, insulin resistance potentiates lipolysis of triglycerides by the hormone-sensitive lipase [34]. This generates the most free fatty acid (FFA) flux in the liver in NAFLD [35]. Insulin resistance in skeletal muscle as a result leads to reduced uptake of glucose, on the other hand in the liver, insulin resistance enhances gluconeogenesis [36]. Iron and NAFLD-resultant compensatory hyperinsulinemia and relative hyperglycaemia promote hepatic de novo lipogenesis and cholesterol synthesis and reduced catabolism of FFA by oxidation [37]. Oxidative stress is considered an important contributor to the pathogenesis of NASH [38]. Excess hepatic iron can promote oxidative stress via Fenton's reaction and is proposed to be a cofactor in the development of NASH.

The regulatory mechanisms of hepcidin have been investigated in animal models, and only a few studies have investigated the role of hepcidin in human NAFLD patients [39]. Hepcidin is an important regulator of liver inflammation [19], and along with its key role in iron homeostasis, it could play a vital part in NASH pathogenesis. It was hypothesised that hepcidin and/or its upstream regulatory factors play a key role in the progression of NAFL to NASH [40]. The elevated hepcidin in NASH seems to be either a reflection of hepatocellular inflammation or simply indicating the induced hepcidin in the early stage of NASH. Hepcidin expression actually appears to be directly enhanced by insulin and down-regulated under insulin resistance, suggesting a possible mechanism for iron loading as an early event in the pathogenesis of NAFLD and T2DM. These findings have raised numerous questions and have stimulated exciting clinical research. With that in mind, it is difficult to predict what additional surprises will emerge from the ongoing study of this fascinating viewpoint.

The elevated ferritin and low expression of hepatic inflammatory cytokines (IL-6; 8-fold, NFNB; 5-fold and IL-1E; 4-fold) in patients with NAFLD with hepatic iron deposition could probably be suggestive of the notion that in this cohort, increased hepcidin expression is more likely attributable to hepatic iron deposition rather than inflammation.

Hepatic HAMP gene expression is induced in patients with NASH compared to that in patients with NAFLD, and presumably, in response to excess hepatic iron in NAFLD patients with iron overload. Two possible mechanisms for hepcidin expression in patients with NASH are likely IL-6-mediated stimulation of JAK2/STAT3 pathway, which results in upregulation of HIF1D. Furthermore, increased hepatic *STAT3* gene expression in NASH patients relative to that in NAFLD patients lends support to this putative hypothesis.

The presence of iron deposition in livers of patients with NAFLD can be classified as hepatocellular, reticuloendothelial or both. A study of 849 adult biopsy specimens performed in the United States showed that reticuloendothelial patterns of iron deposition were associated with advanced fibrosis compared with hepatocellular iron patterns. Biopsy specimens with reticuloendothelial iron were also more likely to have definite steatohepatitis [41]. However, an Italian study on 587 patients with NAFLD found that hepatocellular rather than reticuloendothelial iron was associated with an increased likelihood of liver fibrosis [42].

The reason for the discordant results might be explained by the differences in the patient populations; the subjects in the US study were more ethnically diverse and had higher body mass indices and more advanced fibrosis than those in the Italian study. Interactions between iron metabolism and NAFLD are complex and complicated under active investigation by various researchers. In conclusion, they observed that HAMP expression is elevated in NASH patients and in NAFLD patients with hepatic iron deposits. Their data allowed them to study the interdependence of various regulatory signals such as hepatic iron stores, inflammation and hypoxia or oxidative/ER stress on the expression of hepcidin and inflammatory cytokines. Increased hepcidin expression, which attempts to sequester excess iron, thereby reducing oxidative stress, maybe a protective response.

Bekri et al. showed that hepcidin levels are increased in the adipose tissue of severely obese patients compared with those in the liver, suggesting that severe obesity itself causes hypoferremia due to the overproduction of hepcidin in the adipocytes [43].

Asian Indians are neither associated with iron overload nor with *HFE* gene mutations [44].

The authors suggested that hyperferritinemia in NASH is a non-specific effect of hepatic necroinflammation, reflecting its function as an acute phase protein as a result. Serum ferritin is known to increase because of released from damaged hepatocytes. The authors also previously concluded that serum ferritin levels reflect oxidative stress as well as hepatic iron concentrations and hepatocyte damage in chronic liver disease [45]. Elevated serum ferritin in NASH may be caused by iron-unrelated oxidative stress, such as that derived from FFA, lipid peroxide, cytokines and induction of cytochrome P450 enzymes (CYP2E1 and CYP4AC-) [46]. Thus, the role of hepatic iron in the pathogenesis of NASH or abnormal iron indices in NASH remains debatable and unsettled.

Under usual conditions, intracellular protection from iron-induced oxidative stress is facilitated by sequestration of iron within ferritin [47]. Pathologic states of iron overload often led to saturation of the serum iron transporter, transferrin, which increases the serum levels of toxic non-transferrin bound iron (NTBI). NTBI is readily absorbed by tissues such as the liver and cardiac muscle [48]. The association between hyperferritinemia, insulin resistance and T2DM is compelling. The odds ratios for developing diabetes in those with elevated serum ferritin levels were high at 3.61 for women and 4.94 for men [49–51]. The connotation between hyperferritinemia and histologic markers of liver injury in NAFLD is reasonably firm. In 2004, Bugianesi et al. [43] showed that serum ferritin concentration is not associated with hepatic iron concentration in NAFLD, but is a marker of severe histologic damage.

In an earlier study by Chitturi et al. [44] of 93 patients with NASH, 33% of whom had advanced fibrosis, the authors found that serum ferritin concentration was not an independent predictor of advanced fibrosis. This implies that the ferritin association with NAFLD is not simply a result of NAFLD itself causing hyperferritinemia. Moreover, the results suggest that the link between hyperferritinemia and NAFLD could be explained by insulin resistance. It also appears that it has a direct role in the activation of hepatic macrophages and HSCs. In humans with NAFLD, reticuloendothelial iron has been shown to be associated with apoptosis, indicated by increased serum cytokeratin-18 (CK-18) fragments and increased hepatic TUNEL staining of liver sections [52]. Iron may also contribute to liver injury in NAFLD by generating endoplasmic reticulum stress [53]. Additionally, hepatic iron loading in mice up-regulates cholesterol biosynthesis pathways; this has been proposed as an additional mechanism of iron-induced liver injury in NASH [54].

3. Deteriorative effects of iron against NASH/NAFLD

Iron overload is one of the important risk factors for diabetes. The relationship between iron and diabetes was first recognised in pathologic conditions – namely hereditary hemochromatosis and thalassemia – but high levels of dietary iron also enhance the risk of diabetes. It is generally recognised that iron plays a direct and causal role in diabetes pathogenesis, mediated both by β-cell failure and insulin resistance.

Iron is capable of generating hydroxyl radicals from peroxide and can also inhibit antioxidant defences such as SOD2 [55]. Highly elevated iron levels have been linked to oxidative damage to DNA, lipids and proteins that, in turn, have been implicated in cardiovascular disease, diabetes, atherosclerosis and neurological degeneration, as seen in Alzheimer's disease [56].

Iron homeostatic pathways are tightly associated with inflammatory stressors. Inflammation causes significant upregulation of hepcidin, largely through interleukin-6 (IL-6), and results in large increases in serum ferritin levels.

There is a greater prevalence of iron deficiency in obese (39%) and overweight (12%) children and adolescents than in normal-weight children, the prevalence of iron deficiency in whom is only 4% [28]. The association of iron deficiency with obesity has been confirmed in other populations, which include children and adults of both sexes [57]. The conceivable cases for causality, in turn, can be made in both directions: normal or high iron stores might be required to support higher rates of fatty acid oxidation so that iron-deficient individuals are less able to mobilise and use high fat, or, conversely, the inflammatory nature of obesity might trigger increased hepcidin levels, which limit the absorption of dietary iron.

In the progression of diabetes, ROS can cause both β-cell failure and insulin resistance. β-cells are particularly sensitive to ROS because of low expression of antioxidants such as catalase and SOD2, overexpression of which has been associated with increased β-cell viability [58]. ROS can cause β-cell dysfunction by multiple mechanisms including decreased insulin gene expression secondary to decreased expression of transcription factors necessary for β-cell differentiation, maintenance and insulin gene transcription.

ROS have also been reported to directly affect circulating human insulin by hydroxylation of phenylalanine residues that result in lower affinity binding to the insulin receptor [59]. Finally, ROS can induce insulin resistance through multiple mechanisms; for example, through the activation of FOXO1, which prevents downregulation of gluconeogenesis even in the presence of insulin signalling [60]. Hypoxia-inducible factors 1 and 2 (HIF-1 and HIF-2) regulate cellular responses against low oxygen by upregulating transcription of a diverse set of proteins involved in angiogenesis, erythropoiesis and glycolytic flux [61]. HIFs also regulate iron metabolism, and under conditions of low iron levels, HIF-2 upregulates DMT-1 and DCYTB, whereas HIF-1 upregulates DMT-1 and decreases ferritin [62]. Conversely, cellular iron levels regulate HIF protein levels through the control of prolyl hydroxylase (PHD) activity [63].

Emerging data demonstrate that iron plays an important role in metabolic regulation and the pathophysiology of diabetes. Iron overload is common in T2DM [64, 65]. On the contrary, iron depletion seems to be protective for the development of diabetes. Rats with iron-deficiency anaemia are more insulin sensitive than controls [66], and phlebotomy improves the insulin sensitivity and glycemia, both in nondiabetic subjects [67] and T2DM subjects with high ferritin [68]. These studies suggest that iron plays an important role both in the development and improvement of diabetes. However, the precise molecular mechanisms of iron-associated diabetes are not well understood at present [69].

4. Ameliorating effects of 'hepcidin inducer Laennec and Porcine' for the progression of NASH/NAFLD

NASH is a severe form of fatty liver disease that is defined by the presence of inflammation and fibrosis, ultimately leading to cirrhosis and hepatocellular carcinoma. Shindo et al. [62] evaluated the effect of human placenta extract (HPE) and Laennec treatment in a mouse model of NASH. In the methionine- and choline-deficient (MCD) diet-induced liver injury model, fibrosis started in the regions around the sinusoids.

They dispensed the MCD diet with high-salt loading (add 8% NaCl in the drinking water) to mice deficient in the vasoprotective molecule RAMP2 for 5 weeks, with or without HPE. In both the HPE and control groups, fibrosis was observed in regions adjacent to the sinusoids, but fibrosis was not so pronounced in the HPE-treated mice. Levels of TNF-α and MMP9 expression were also significantly reduced in

HPE-treated mice, and oxidative stress was suppressed in the perivascular region. These observations indicate that HPE ameliorates NASH-associated pathologies by suppressing inflammation, oxidative stress and liver fibrosis.

HPE has been prescribed clinically to treat chronic hepatitis, liver cirrhosis and other hepatic diseases for more than 40 years in Japan. In an experimental animal model of hepatitis, HPE reportedly ameliorated hepatic injury through liver regeneration and inhibition of inflammatory reactions and hepatocyte apoptosis [70, 71]. Moreover, Shimokobe et al. recently reported that HPE is effective in NASH patients who were unresponsive to lifestyle intervention [72].

As for histopathological changes in the liver, silver staining histological sample revealed fibrotic areas adjacent to the sinusoids in both groups; however, the fibrosis was not so severe in HPE-treated mice. By using immunofluorescent staining, the authors observed high expression levels of p67 phox, a cytosolic component of NADPH oxidase, in the perivascular regions of all mice; however, the expression levels were less marked in HPE-treated mice. Levels of 4HNE, a lipid peroxidation product, were also decreased in HPE-treated mice. Judging from these observations, it is indicated that HPE treatment for ameliorated liver injury is possible by reducing inflammation, oxidative stress and fibrosis.

In an earlier study, HPE was shown to suppress inflammation in a chronic arthritis rat model using complete Freund's adjuvant [73]. Direct effects of HPE on the production of pro-inflammatory cytokines and mediators have also been reported. For example, HPE reportedly inhibits the production of nitric oxide, TNF-α and cyclooxygenase-2 in lipopolysaccharide-stimulated RAW264.7 macrophages [74]. In the present study, the authors found that HPE significantly suppressed TNF-α expression in an MCD fed-diet model. This suggests that HPE may suppress the progression of chronic inflammation initiated by lipid accumulation within hepatocytes of the NASH patients.

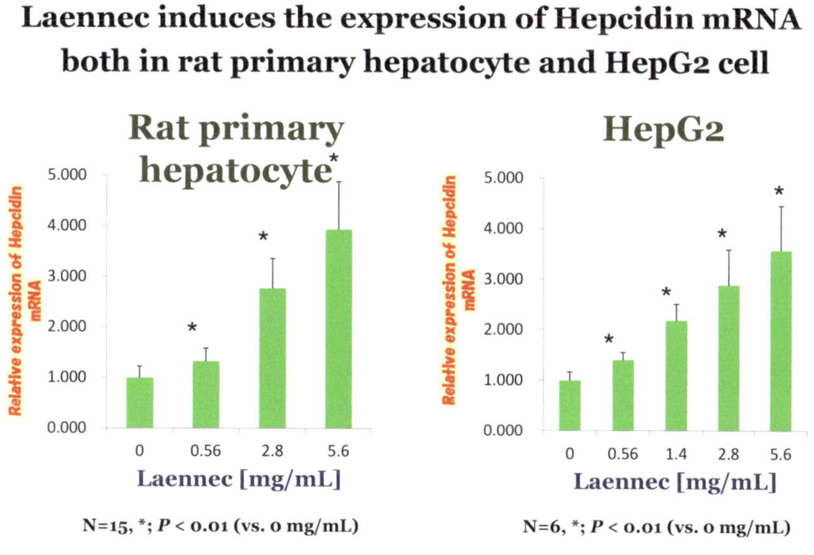

Figure 1.
The most important basic data is expressed. Laennec induces the expression of hepcidin mRNA both in rat primary hepatocyte and HepG2 cells in a dose dependent manner; this means that in the human body, the possibility of hepcidin mediated action of Laennec might be the main route or at least one of the important mechanism of its efficacy in regulating iron metabolism.

Besides inflammation, oxidative stress seems to also contribute to chronic liver injury. In that regard, HPE showed both anti-oxidative and anti-inflammatory activities in rats exposed to benzopyrene (BaP) [75]. Application of H_2O_2 to cultured cells is performed to evaluate the cellular damage caused by oxidative stress. It is also observed that serum hepcidin levels are typically elevated in individuals with NASH [76]. As this in itself fails to explain iron loading in NASH, one might consider that dysregulated iron metabolism occurs in NASH independently of hepcidin.

The contribution of adipose tissue-derived hepcidin to the serum hepcidin pool is uncertain, however, this is another potential factor that may explain the increased serum hepcidin levels in NASH. Further complexity in these relationships arises when one considers that iron deficiency has been shown to be associated with obesity, and in women with obesity and NAFLD [77, 78]. Together, these findings suggest that the interaction between iron and lipid metabolism is multi-faceted. It seems that 'just enough' but 'not too much' iron may be critical for preventing dysfunctional lipid metabolism.

Previous studies [73–75] have revealed that the administration of Laennec significantly improved T2DM complicated with NASH and other chronic liver diseases, suggesting the importance of iron regulation on insulin-resistant T2DM showing hyperferritinemia.

Thus, more experimental and clinical studies are required to confirm or refute the claim that hepcidin has a rolc in T2DM. To shed light on the factors that alter hepcidin expression, the authors performed experiments with HepG2 and HuH7, human hepatoma cell lines that are widely used for this purpose. Despite the considerable advances made recently, further explorations are required to investigate the cellular mechanisms and functions of peripheral hepcidin, as well as its regulation in different organs (**Figures 1** and **2**).

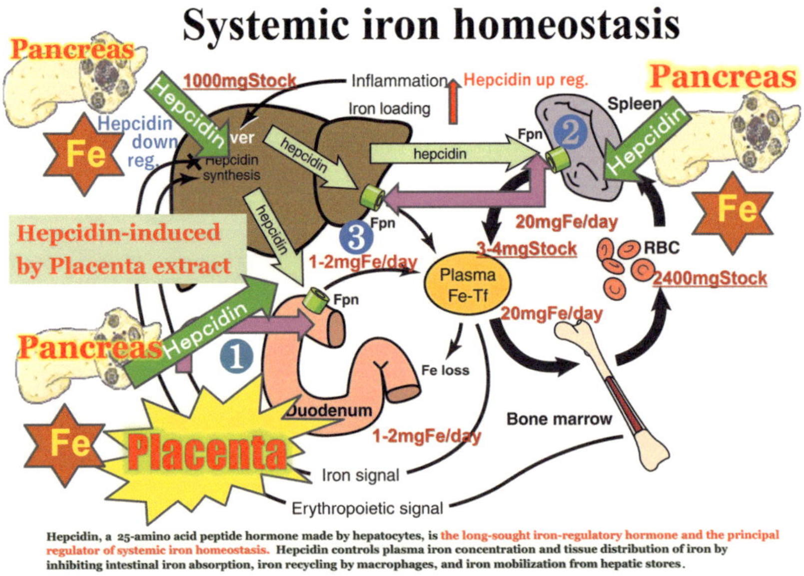

Ganz T et al. JASN 2007;18:394-400 modified

Figure 2.
Systemic iron homeostasis is regulated by hepcidin. Judging from the clinical data of Laennec, formerly obtained through the treatment of chronic liver diseases such as NASH and chronic hepatitis type C, the sites of action of Laennec resemble those of hepcidin. Hepcidin is also expressed in the pancreas of rats and humans, which means that pancreas is an iron-regulating organ beyond their proper glucose–regulatory function. According to basic data, the regulation of hepcidin expression is similar in the liver and in the endocrine pancreas.

5. Placenta-derived drugs Laennec (i.v) and Porcine (oral) are capable of improving T2DM complicating with NASH/NAFLD through the action of 'hepcidin inducer'

The discovery of hepcidin and its role in iron metabolism could lead to novel therapies for hereditary hemochromatosis and other iron-loading diseases. Laennec (parenteral) and Porcine (oral), which are hepcidin inducers, actually improved iron overload in a hereditary hemochromatosis patient, without performing sequential phlebotomy. This suggests the possibility of not only improving the prognosis of hereditary hemochromatosis but also ameliorating complications, such as type 2 diabetes, liver fibrosis and hypogonadism. Laennec and Porcine can completely replace continuous venesection in patients with hereditary hemochromatosis and may improve other iron-overloading disorders caused by hepcidin deficiency and/or insufficiency [73, 75] (**Figures 1–4**).

The association with hepcidin is supposed in many kinds of human diseases, furthermore, most of these diseases are influenced by alterations in hepcidin concentrations [73, 76]. Hepcidin-targeted therapies may improve the manifestations and biochemical abnormalities of patients with iron disorders. Although no specific hepcidin therapies are currently available, several compounds are under development as hepcidin agonists or antagonists [77]. Moreover, hepcidin either has a primary or a secondary role in insulin resistance, which is a characteristic of T2DM. However, it remains inconclusive whether serum hepcidin levels are an independent risk factor in the etiopathogenesis of T2DM. By inducing preferable and appropriate amounts of hepcidin, placenta-derived drugs could improve the clinical course of NASH complicated with T2DM and hyperferritinemia by attenuating

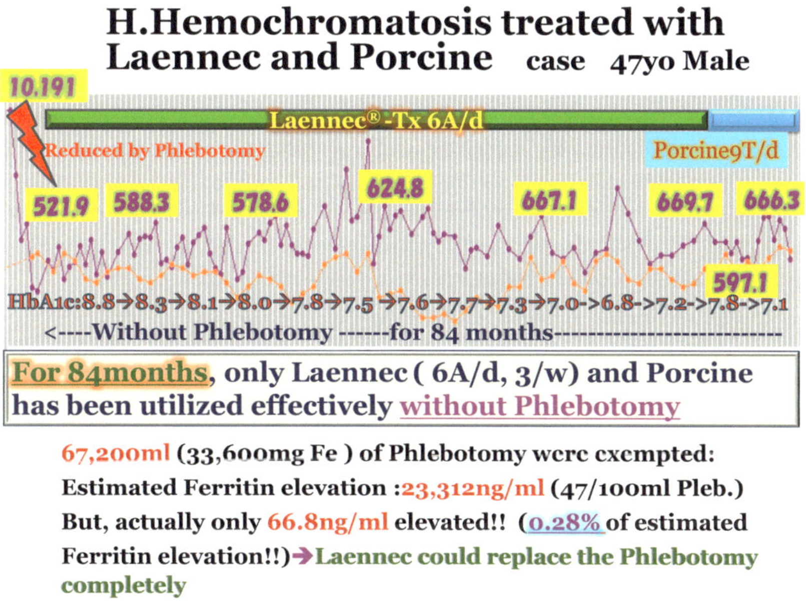

Figure 3.
H. hemochromatosis treated with Laennec and porcine. Case, 47-year-old male. For 74 months, only Laennec (6A/d, 3/w) and porcine have been utilised effectively without phlebotomy. 67,200 ml (33,600 mg Fe) of phlebotomy were exempted: Estimated ferritin elevation 23,312 ng/ml (47/100 ml phlebotomy). Actually only 66.8 ng/ml elevated (0.28% of estimated ferritin elevation).

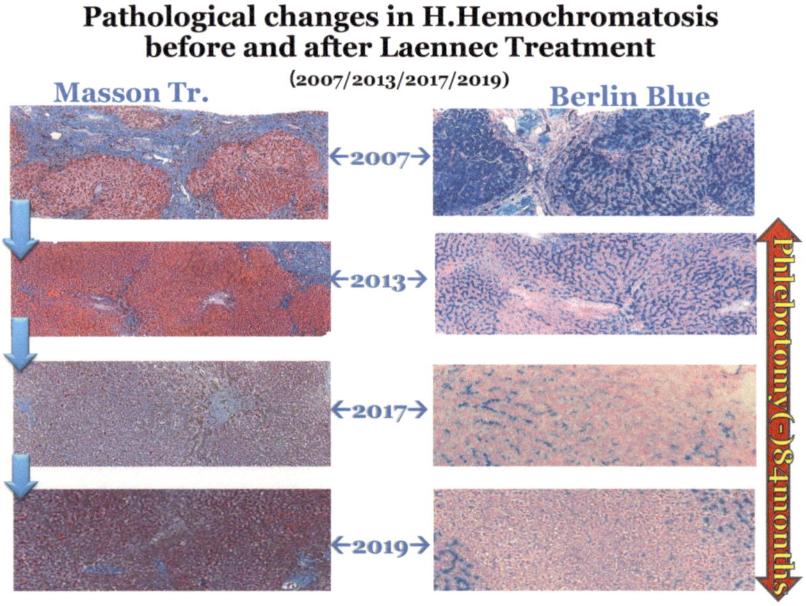

Figure 4.
After treatment with Laennec without phlebotomy for 84 months, the histological evaluation revealed a remarkable reduction in iron deposition and fibrosis. At the same time, remarkable improvements in the quality of life (QOL) and erectile dysfunction (ED) were observed. During these periods, oral administration with porcine was replaced with Laennec for 8 months; however, the efficacy remained the same.

the iron-induced oxidative stress and iron accumulation in both hepatocytes and pancreatic β-cells [78].

It is generally confirmed that iron overload causes insulin deficiency by promoting pancreatic β-cell apoptosis. Because of their stringent dependence on mitochondrial glucose metabolism and their limited antioxidant capacity [79], β-cells are extremely susceptible to oxidative stress. Through their divalent metal transporter, pancreatic β-cells can avariciously take up non-Tf-bound iron [80], which can promote oxidative stress by catalysing the Fenton reaction. Elevated iron levels oxidise various biomolecules, such as nucleic acids, proteins, and lipids, which may contribute to the development of T2DM by decreasing the insulin secretion from pancreatic β-cells, with a concomitant increase in insulin resistance [14, 76].

In our clinical data: Laennec has been administered [73] (**Figures 3** and **4**) to a patient with hereditary hemochromatosis without phlebotomy. HbA1c levels have further improved by Laennec treatment (more than 2% declined) for 84 months without changing the medications for diabetes treatment. These results are probably due to the additive efficacy of Laennec in reducing iron-originated ROS, enhancing the anti-inflammatory action with concomitant improvement in liver fibrosis, and diminishing the iron deposition in hepatocytes. Laennec was also administered to patients with NASH with T2DM (**Figures 5–8**); treatment with Laennec significantly improved the T2DM, reduced the serum ferritin level, and decreased the iron deposition in the hepatocytes [73, 74]. The regulation of iron and glucose metabolism is possibly due to the pancreatic β-cells' ability to co-release insulin and hepcidin.

The data published by Kulaksiz et al. [81] demonstrated that hepcidin is expressed in the pancreas of rats and humans. Further analysis showed that it was localised in the β-cells of the islets of Langerhans. In addition, in vitro experiments performed

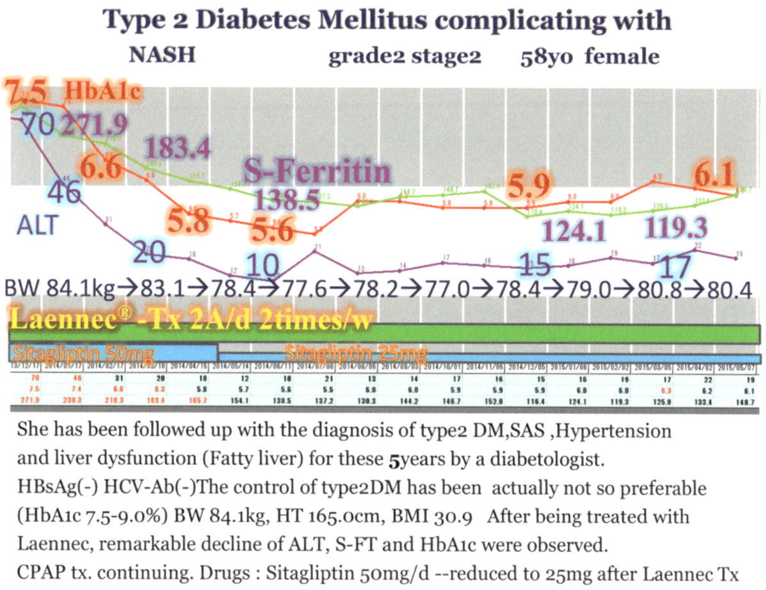

Figure 5.
Type 2 diabetes mellitus complicating with NASH grade 2, stage 2, 58 years old female. H.P.I: she has been followed up with the diagnosis of type 2 DM, SAS, hypertension and liver dysfunction (fatty liver) for these 5 years by a diabetologist. HBsAg (−) HCV (−) the control type 2 DM has been actually not so preferable (HbA1c 7.5–9.0%) BW 84.1 kg, HT 84.1 kg, HT 165.0 cm, BMI 30.9. As for SAS: CPAP tx continuing drugs for DM: sitagliptin 50 mg/d reduced to 25 mg after Laennec Tx.

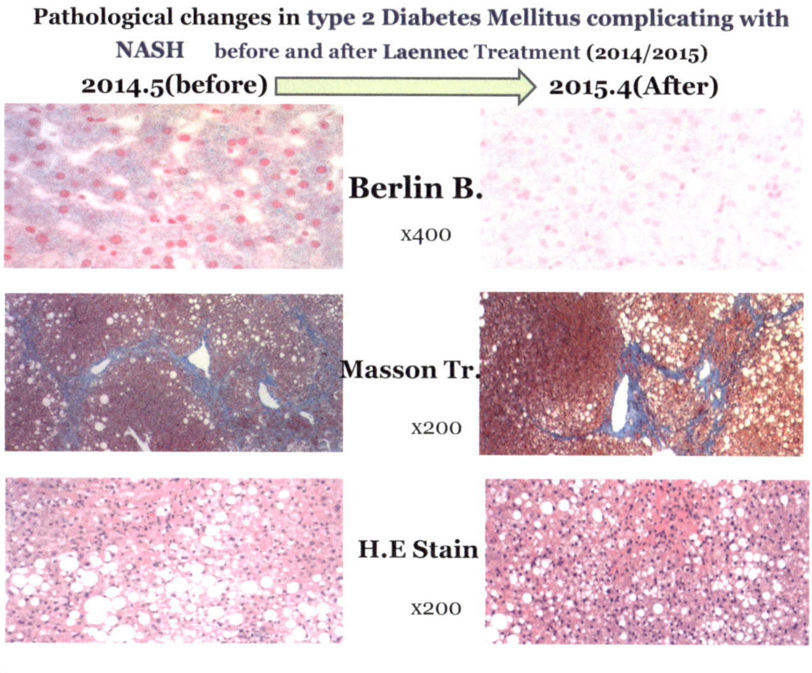

Figure 6.
The histological evaluation revealed the presence of fatty metamorphosis, inflammation, pericellular fibrosis, ballooning of hepatocyte, Mallory body and iron deposition mainly in the hepatocyte. After treating with Laennec, the histological evaluation revealed remarkable improvement in iron deposition and fibrosis, as well as amelioration of inflammation and fatty metamorphosis.

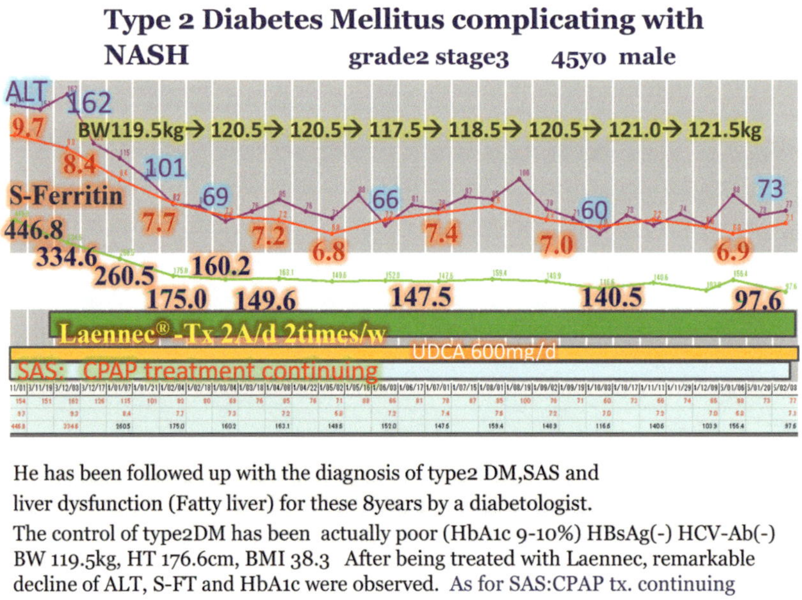

Figure 7.

Type 2 diabetes mellitus complicating with NASH grade 2, stage 3, 45 years old male. H.P.I: he has been followed up with the diagnosis of type 2 DM, SAS and liver dysfunction (fatty liver) for these 8 years by a diabetologist. The control of type 2 DM has been actually poor (HbA1c 9–10%) HBsAg (−) HCV-ab (−) BW 119.5 kg, HT 176.6 cm, BMI 38.3. As for SAS: CPAP tx continuing drugs for DM: [1] metformin 2250 mg/d [2] sitagliptin 100 mg/d [3] gliclazide 40 mg/d.

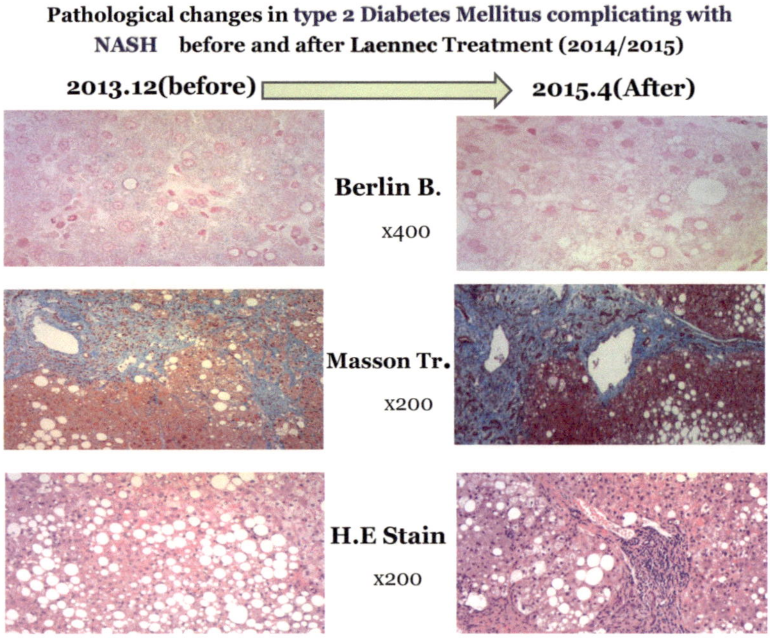

Figure 8.

Histological evaluation revealed the presence of fatty metamorphosis, inflammation, pericellular fibrosis and iron deposition in the hepatocyte. After treating with Laennec, the histological evaluation revealed remarkable improvement in iron deposition and fibrosis as well as amelioration of inflammation and fatty metamorphosis. In addition to these pathological changes, remarkable improvements in biochemical data and QOL were observed.

in this study demonstrated that hepcidin expression in β-cells is directly regulated by iron. Iron is important for normal insulin secretion. However, excessive amounts of iron can affect β-cell function in hemochromatosis models [82–84], causing iron accumulation in the islets, a reduction in insulin secretion and an increase in the apoptosis of β-cells. In contrast, a reduction in the iron pool was shown to protect against diabetes and loss of β-cell function in an obese (ob/ob) mouse model [85]. These observations suggest that hepcidin produced by β-cells may be involved in the intrinsic regulation of pancreatic iron and glucose homeostasis [22].

In accordance with this study, the possibility of replacing phlebotomy with placenta-derived drugs, Laennec and Porcine, was evidenced through the pharmacological mechanism of inducing hepcidin production and suppressing iron-related oxidative stress [86]. Furthermore, these results strongly suggest that Laennec and Porcine are considerably effective not only for H.H but also for other iron loading diseases, such as β-thalassemia, MDS, NASH complicated with T2DM, and autoimmune liver disease [primary biliary cirrhosis (PBC) and autoimmune hepatitis (AIH)] [73–75]. The efficacy of removing iron from the liver will improve the prognosis of patients with these types of iron-loading hepatic disorders. Thus, more experimental and clinical studies are required to confirm the claim that hepcidin plays an important role in chronic liver diseases and complicating T2DM [87]. These are promising drugs that can suppress iron-induced oxidative injury as well as iron deposition in multiple organs, which will improve the prognosis of patients who developed iron-overloading disorders (**Figures 5–8**) [73–75].

In addition, in some types of β-thalassemia (especially intermediate), inducing hepcidin by administering Laennec and Porcine can improve the iron-overloading conditions in these patients without affecting the underlying cause of their haemolytic anaemia.

In general, serum hepcidin levels are typically elevated in individuals with NASH [68]. As this in itself fails to explain the cause of iron loading in NASH, one might consider that dysregulated iron metabolism occurs in NASH independently of hepcidin. One of the possible mechanisms by which hepcidin inducer Laennec is capable of improving iron metabolism in NAFLD/NASH might be the induction of the alternative route of hepcidin, which might be relevant in the progression of NAFLD/NASH. Furthermore, there might be some kind of 'hepcidin resistance' in NAFLD/NASH patients, which is observed in T2DM patients as 'insulin resistance'.

In conclusion, the present study suggests that s-ferritin elevation in our patients is a marker of metabolic syndrome with hepatic steatosis and insulin resistance and not of iron overload. The direct pathogenic mechanism, however, remains unknown. In the absence of in vivo data, any iron-independent role of hepcidin in the host defence remains speculative.

6. Laennec and Porcine also have the effects of anti-inflammation and immune modulation in the treatment of chronic liver diseases

For the clinician, the serum elevation of ferritin in chronic liver diseases (CLD), with the exception of hemochromatosis, is always assumed to be a non-specific marker of hepatic inflammation and not of iron overload [88]. It is generally considered that iron is a putative component that interacts with oxygen radicals, and high rates of hyperferritinemia together with increased hepatic iron stores have been demonstrated in NASH [22].

In the progression and pathogenesis of NASH, the role of hepatic iron still remains debatable. It is empirically accepted that iron-restricted diets or phlebotomy reduce hepatic damage as well as insulin resistance (IR) in patients with NAFLD/NASH [89]. However, the exact mechanisms involved in iron accumulation in NASH remain unresolved. Several mechanisms such as dysregulation of iron-regulatory molecules, genetic factors linked to IR and erythrophagocytosis by Kupffer cells might be responsible for hepatic iron overload in NASH [90].

A simple clinical study of phlebotomy treatment was reported by Chakraberti and Adams, performed on a series of 56 patients with histology-proven NAFLD [91]. Liver biopsy and liver iron concentration (LIC) were evaluated at entry and 6 months after phlebotomy. They did not find any significant correlation between hepatic inflammation as measured by NAS score, LIC and the level of serum ferritin and other genetic markers of inflammation, such as ESR and CRP. The authors had the conclusion that elevated serum ferritin is associated with hepatic iron accumulation, but that liver inflammation is not the cause of increased serum ferritin in patients with NAFLD.

Recently, other authors [92] demonstrated that elevated ferritin levels reflect iron stores, and not hepatic inflammation, being predictors of vascular damage in NAFLD. Irrespective of the underlying mechanisms, the only certainty is that an increased serum ferritin level in NAFLD is not a marker or a cause of inflammation, but a consequence of iron accumulation within the hepatocyte.

The resident macrophages in the sinusoids of the liver, Kupffer cells, have been widely implicated in hepatic injury such as endotoxin–mediated liver injury. Kupffer cells are known to express the death ligands, tumour necrosis factor α (TNF α), TNF-related apoptosis-inducing ligand (TRAIL), and Fas ligand [93, 94].

As a consequence of chronic tissue damage, HSCs, as well as other extracellular matrices – producing cells such as fibroblasts and myofibroblasts – undergo a process of activation towards a phenotype characterised by increased proliferation, motility, contractility and synthesis of extracellular matrix components. HSC activation is regulated by several soluble factors, including cytokines, chemokines, growth factors and products of oxidative stress as well as by extensive changes in composition and organisation of extracellular matrix components. Controlled cell death (apoptosis) could also be a mechanism underlying the termination of HSC proliferation. Spontaneous apoptosis is detected in parallel with HSC activation. Hepatic fibrosis is a complex dynamic process mediated by the death of hepatocytes and the activation of HSCs. Lipid peroxidation including the generation of ROS, TGF-β and TNF-α can be implicated as a cause of hepatic fibrosis.

The major source of ROS production in hepatocytes is NADH and NADPH oxidases localised in mitochondria. NADH and NADPH oxidases leak ROS as part of their operation. Hepatic fibrosis itself causes no symptoms but can lead to end-stage cirrhosis. In cirrhosis, the failure to properly replaced destroyed hepatocytes and the excessive collagen deposition to distort blood flow through the liver (portal hypertension) results in severe liver dysfunction.

Under physiological conditions, hydrogen peroxide plays an important role in intracellular signalling. In terms of pathological actions, ROS participate in the development of liver diseases. In this situation, hydrogen peroxide is converted into the hydroxyl radical, which is a harmful and highly reactive ROS, in the presence of transition metals such as iron. At the cellular levels, origin of hepatic fibrosis is initiated by the damage of hepatocytes, followed by the accumulation of neutrophils and macrophages including Kupffer cells on the sites of injury and inflammation in the liver. When hepatocytes are continuously damaged, leading to cell death, the production of extracellular matrix proteins such as collagens predominates over hepatocellular regeneration. Overproduced collagens are deposited in injured areas instead of destroyed hepatocytes.

Judging from our clinical data presented before [73–75], Laennec and Porcine could have improved chr. liver diseases (CHC, NASH, PBC, AIH etc.) through the mechanisms of anti-inflammatory and immune modulative actions, which were evidenced through the fundamental examinations performed by Shindo et al. [62].

7. Heterogeneity of NASH/NAFLD from the viewpoints of etiopathogenic backgrounds and their sensitivity to each treatment procedure.

NAFLD, the most common chronic liver disease in the United States, European and Asian countries is an extremely heterogeneous disorder in its etiopathogenic backgrounds and clinical manifestations [95]. The pathogenesis of NAFLD is multifactorial and complicated; thus, several systemic alterations and individual variations have been implicated and discussed [96].

The primary insult of lipid excess is followed by variable contributions from pathogenic drivers, such as lipotoxicity and immune system response with activation; and modifiers, such as genetic susceptibilities, high calory diet, added small amount of alcohol, and dysbiosis. Although there are considerable heterogeneities in NAFLD progression and the development of NASH, only a subset of NAFLD develops into NASH, which is the most unsolved problem and mysterious issue.

Potential explanations for this variability include differences in etiopathogenic drivers [2], dynamic multiphasic progression, constitutional/genetic backgrounds, complicated diseases, biological reactions, metabolic responses, etc. [97].

7.1 With or without 'T2DM and insulin resistance'

Diabetes is highly prevalent in patients with NASH/NAFLD and vice versa.

Three studies using Fibroscan showed that 12–18% of diabetic patients are estimated to have significant liver fibrosis by different cut-offs [98–100]. Decreased levels of HbA1c [101] were more strongly associated with fibrosis improvement in 39 Japanese patients with diabetes and NAFLD who underwent sequential liver biopsies. Thus, these three clinical parameters, including ALT, body weight and HbA1c (ABC), can become the milestones for the treatment of NASH, although the appropriate goal of each parameter to ameliorate hepatic fibrosis will be established in the near future.

In a cross-sectional multicentre study conducted by JSGNAFLD, the presence of diabetes was found to be associated with advanced fibrosis in 1365 biopsy-proven NAFLD patients [102]. 'With or without T2DM' is a crucial problem for treating NAFLD/NASH patients because complicated T2DM itself modulates the clinical manifestations of NAFLD/NASH and affects the sensitivities to treatment procedures and the prognosis of each disease. If some effective treatments are developed and preferable improvement of NAFLD/NASH can be achieved, the control of T2DM will improve unexpectedly. Mounting evidence suggests that more experimental and clinical studies are needed to confirm or refute the claim that hepcidin has a role or relevance with T2DM complicated with NAFLD/NASH.

Recently, attention has been shifting towards the iron regulatory hormone hepcidin and its possible role in the etiopathogenesis of T2DM. Interpreting this critically, notably, hepcidin in the pancreas is expressed exclusively in the islets of Langerhans, which constitute merely a small compartment of the total pancreatic parenchyma. Very likely, the regulation of iron and glucose metabolism is distinctly coupled at least at the pancreatic level by the co-release of insulin and hepcidin [81].

7.2 With or without 'hyperferritinemia and iron overloading, related with T2DM'

A strong correlation between iron overload and several manifestations of the metabolic syndrome including NAFLD and T2DM has been demonstrated recently. It has clashed that increased ferritin levels observed in most patients with NASH are due to the underlying necro-inflammatory condition, which assists the release of tissue iron and ferritin into the blood [103].

The corelation between NASH and IR has recently been weaved as a 'new iron overload syndrome' characterised by hyperferritinemia. The dysmetabolic iron overload syndrome has now been established as a frequent finding in the general population, occurring in about one-third of patients with NAFLD and metabolic syndrome. Altered regulation of iron transport genetic factors is considered to be the main contributor to iron overload [26]. The exact mechanisms underlying the deposition of hepatic iron remain unknown and unsettled. One of the clinical factors associated with steatosis, IR and subclinical inflammation, often in the presence of predisposing features of NASH, is the build-up of iron in the liver accompanied by increased levels of serum ferritin, which is highly suggestive of the central role of iron in disease progression [104].

Iron is known to generate highly reactive hydroxyl radicals through the Fenton reaction, and the resultant ROS may contribute to liver damage. Significant increases in hepatic 8-OHdG generated by OH radicals have been reported in patients with NASH, particularly in correlation with iron overload, IR and severity of hepatic steatosis [26]. The mechanisms involved in iron accumulation in NAFLD, and in inducing IR, metabolic, hepatic and vascular damage by iron accumulation are not yet well understood and should be further investigated [92].

The association between hyperferritinemia, insulin resistance and T2DM has been discussed among hepatologists, diabetologists and endocrinologists recently. There is an increased prevalence of T2DM associated with two common iron overload conditions, HFE hereditary hemochromatosis (HH) and β-thalassemia major [28]. The persistence of the association between serum ferritin concentration and T2DM after correction for hsCRP implies that inflammation alone does not entirely explain the association between hyperferritinemia and diabetes.

Bugianesi et al. [43] found that the serum ferritin concentration is not associated with hepatic iron concentration in NAFLD but is a marker of severe histologic damage in 2004. In the large NASH Clinical Research Network (CRN) cohort of 628 patients, Kowdley et al. [105] demonstrated that a serum ferritin concentration greater than 1.5 times the upper limit of normal was independently associated with advanced fibrosis and increased NAFLD activity score. However, other studies have not found such a clear association [39, 106].

Notably, in an Italian cohort of 587 patients with NAFLD, Valenti et al. [26] showed that serum ferritin concentration did not predict fibrosis stage >1. As would be expected, the serum ferritin concentration was higher in the patients who had hepatic iron staining than those who did not, but those with non-parenchymal iron had much higher ferritin values (606 μg/L) than those with hepatocellular iron (serum ferritin 354 μg/L) $P < 0.0001$. This suggests that macrophage iron can cause hyperferritinemia either by direct release of ferritin or cytokine-mediated stimulation of ferritin released by other cells.

Moreover, these results tend to suggest that the link between hyperferritinemia and NAFLD could be explained by insulin resistance. In NAFLD pathogenesis, the role of hepatic iron has largely focused on the generation of oxidative stress by iron. Considering oxidative stress is an established key component of NASH pathogenesis [107], the role of iron mediating liver injury in NAFLD via this mechanism has been well studied. Oxidative stress leads to cell death via depletion of ATP, NAD and glutathione, and by direct damage to DNA, lipids and proteins within hepatocytes in NASH. Furthermore, oxidative stress leads to an increase in the production of pro-inflammatory cytokines and fibrogenic responses. Not only does oxidative stress potentiate steatohepatitis, characterised by inflammation and cell death, but it can also increase steatosis by preventing the secretion of very low-density lipoprotein (VLDL) through increased degradation of apolipoprotein B100 (ApoB100) [108].

In conclusion, iron has been gradually recognised as a regulator of adipose tissue function. There are definite pieces of evidence which support the role of iron in the regulation of adipose tissue inflammation, adipokine regulation and adipose tissue lipolysis. At present, most pieces of evidence support the role of adipose tissue iron in the pathogenesis of insulin resistance and T2DM, although clearly, these mechanisms may be highly relevant in NAFLD.

It has been suggested that elevated serum ferritin is associated with several metabolic disorders. However, no reported study has assessed the association between serum ferritin and sarcopenia despite the close relationship between sarcopenia and metabolic disorders.

The question then arises whether the concentration of hepcidin in T2DM subjects is primary or secondary to elevated body iron stores. This might be an important assignment to find a key to the settlement of the dispute.

7.3 With or without 'iron deposition in hepatocyte and/or Kupffer cell'

Although iron is indispensable for normal physiology and biochemical reactions, excess iron is toxic and harmful because it can accelerate the Fenton reaction that generates noxious reactive oxygen species (ROS) and severely damages cells and tissues in the human body. Thus, maintenance of body iron homeostasis is pivotal, particularly because there is no physiological pathway for removal of excessive iron from the body [109]. Systemic iron regulation is mediated via the liver-secreted iron regulating hormone hepcidin under normal physiological conditions [110]. Several studies have reported the fibrosis-enhancing effects of iron. For instance, induced collagen deposition in gerbil [111], iron elevated collagen gene expression in HSCs and increased TGF-β expression in rats [112], and promoted cirrhosis in mice [113]. Ramm et al. [114] demonstrated the correlation between LIC and HSC-activation in humans, resulting in increased expression of α-SMA and collagen deposition in patients with hemochromatosis for the first time. Similar results were observed in rat HSCs, wherein iron increased HSC-cell proliferation and selectively increased collagen synthesis without affecting non-collagen proteins [115].

In the pathogenesis of NAFLD, iron has been widely implicated, therefore represents a potential target for treatment. Correlations between the serum ferritin concentration and NAFLD are noted in most studies, although serum ferritin is an indistinct measure of iron loading. A large number of mechanisms underlying the pathogenic role of hepatic iron in NAFLD have been demonstrated in animal and cell culture models. However, the human data linking hepatic iron to liver injury in NAFLD is not so clear, with seemingly conflicting evidence, supporting either an effect of iron in hepatocytes or within reticuloendothelial cells. Adipose tissue has emerged as a key site where iron may have a pathogenic role in NAFLD [116].

An investigation of the serum ferritin level and histological findings including iron deposition in 628 patients with NAFLD was performed by Kowdley et al. [105]. This large cross-sectional study revealed that elevated serum ferritin (>1.5 × UNL) was associated with advanced hepatic fibrosis (odds ratio [OR], 1.66; 95% confidence interval [CI], 1.05–2.62; P = 0.028) and a higher NAS (OR, 1.99; 95% CI, 1.06–3.75; P = 0.033). Elevated serum ferritin levels (seen in approximately 20% of the subjects) were associated with greater iron accumulation in the body (i.e., a high serum iron and transferrin-iron saturation) and greater hepatic iron deposition in both the reticuloendothelial system and hepatocytes.

It was also elucidated that the patients with increased serum ferritin levels also had higher serum transaminases and gamma-glutamyl transferase and a lower platelet count. Interestingly, even in patients without a hepatic iron overload on histology, higher serum ferritin was correlated with advanced stage of the disease.

7.4 With or without 'inflammation and elevation of cytokines'

One of modifying factors in NAFLD/NASH is hepatic iron content (HIC) [117]. Iron accumulation exacerbates hepatic oxidative stress and can, therefore, affect susceptibility to oxidant stress induced by fatty acid oxidation [118]. HIC is susceptive to factors that differ among individuals (polymorphisms in genes such as HFE) and factors that might change during the lifetime of individuals, including sex-related factors (menstruation or pregnancy) and diet (consumption of greasy meal, roughage or red meat) [119]. The lipotoxic outcomes of identical fatty acid exposures can, therefore, differ based on complicated factors that modulate hepatic iron content. Inflammation is required to clear damage-related debris and stimulate local accumulation of other wound-healing cells, such as liver progenitors and myofibroblasts. However, excessive inflammation can compromise the viability of residual hepatocytes and promote over-growth of progenitors and myofibroblasts, laying the groundwork for progressive fibrosis to liver cirrhosis and carcinogenesis. Therefore, the liver is variably repopulated with relatively immature or dysfunctional hepatocytes as long as wound-healing responses are active and continuing. This potentiates metabolic stress and increases the risk of liver cancer [120].

Recent studies have suggested several possibilities in progressing liver fibrosis, involving inflammation caused by OS associated with lipid peroxidation, endogenous toxins of fructose metabolites, cytokine activation and NO [9]. Mitochondrial dysfunction not only facilitated the production of ROS but also contributed to the progression of NAFLD by inducing hepatic inflammatory cytokines. The network of obesity, IR and adipokine/cytokine has been hypothesised to induce both liver fat accumulation and NASH development [121]. ROS along with products of lipid peroxidation leads to increased release of several cytokines (tumour necrosis factor-alpha (TNF-α), Fas ligand), which play a key role in cell death, inflammation and fibrosis [107]. Lipid peroxidation, release of inflammatory cytokines and cell death are the consequences of ROS-mediated mechanisms. Biologically active lipid peroxidation products and cytokines take action together by inducing hepatic inflammation, leading to the development of diverse hepatic lesions associated with NASH. The inflammatory response is induced because of the upregulation of pro-inflammatory cytokines including TNF-α, interleukin (IL) 1 and IL-6 [122], which play an essential role in directing polymorpho-and mono-nuclear leukocytes into flamed tissue. The effects of TNF-α in NASH are enhanced through an abnormal cytokine profile and increased expression of the TNF-α-receptor in the liver [123]. This contributes to additional lipid peroxidation of the mitochondrial membranes, thereby worsening their function and further inducing OS [94]. Adipose tissue shows prominent deregulation of genes related to inflammation in patients with NASH. Induction of NADPH oxidase by TNF-α also leads to inflammation through the expression of TNF receptor-1 and activation of nuclear factor kappa B (NF-κB).

In the pathogenesis of steatohepatitis, hepatic inflammation and fibrogenic progression are pivotal features. Although hepatocyte damage and ROS are regarded to be the initial triggers of inflammation, additional factors such as mitochondrial dysfunction and ER stress have also been implicated as contributory factors in the progression of NAFLD to NASH, by promoting generation of signals and mediators of inflammation.

The association of elevated serum iron values and increased hepatic tissue ferritin deposition with hepatic inflammation and IR in patients with NASH have been well established [94]. In contrast, ROS and lipid peroxidation cause direct damage to hepatocytes by affecting membranes, proteins and DNA [124]. The ensuing damage to nuclear and mtDNA results in necro-inflammation, particularly in the nuclei/cytoplasm of hepatocytes and sinusoidal cells.

The results of current research suggest that hepcidin may dampen inflammatory cytokines through a mechanism that is not well understood. Because excessive inflammation is damaging in many infections, the potential role of hepcidin as a mediator of the innate immune response is a new and unexpected area of study.

7.5 With or without 'sleeping apnoea syndrome (SAS), CPAP-Tx (+) or (−)'

Another serious clinical condition in understanding NAFLD/NASH is the presence of obstructive sleep apnoea (OSA), characterised by upper airway obstruction (causing intermittent hypoxia and ROS), and interrupted sleep [125]. Both conditions have been associated together as a cause/result/modifying factor or potential co-occurring complications of obesity and NAFLD/NASH [126, 127].

The two-hits hypothesis is one of the prevalent theories for the development of NASH. This theory indicates that benign hepatic steatosis may be the first hit, and then, another precipitating factor (second hit) may load and progress the pathogenesis of NAFLD/NASH [128]. The involvement of OSA as a second hit in NASH development is evidenced by both experimental and epidemiological reports.

In a mice experiment, Zamora-Valdés and Méndez-Sánchez evidenced that exposure to a high-fat diet along with chronic intermittent hypoxia was associated with lobular inflammation and fibrosis and with significant increases in the hepatic levels of pro-inflammatory cytokines (interleukin 1β and 6 and tumour necrosis factor α), as well as collagen-1α mRNA. Other in vivo experiments showed concordant results [129]. Oxidative stress and the release of hypoxia-inducible factor-1 are hypothesised to be the main players in this association [130].

Concurrently, epidemiological studies have showna higher prevalence of NASH in OSA patients, as well as a higher prevalence of OSA in NASH patients and vice versa. However, the evidence remains largely inconclusive, i.e., some studies have reported significant elevation in serum liver enzymes in OSA patients [131], whereas other studies failed to record such observations [132]. In a sample of 54,169 participants, significant association between NASH and OSA was observed. At the same time, significant associations between NASH and obesity, DM and metabolic syndrome were also observed, indicating the possible involvement of these conditions in the pathogenesis of NASH.

Some convincing mechanisms were speculated to explain this association lately. Oxidative stress remains the predominant hypothesis. This occurs through repetitive cycles of hypoxia/reoxygenation every night, which disturb mitochondrial respiration along with bouts of catecholamine release, inducing metabolic changes [133]. Moreover, hypoxia stimulates fibrosis and angiogenesis by enhancing the expression of hypoxia-inducible factor-1α, vascular endothelial growth factor, angiotensin-I-converting enzyme and transforming growth factor β1 [134].

Furthermore, hypoxia is an established risk factor for inflammation [135]. This study documented a significant association between NASH and other complicating factors such as obesity, DM and metabolic syndrome. The association between NASH and hypertension, obesity and DM shows the full picture of metabolic syndrome. If the NASH patients complicating with SAS could be treated by CPAP appropriately, the more enthusiastically they continue the procedure, the more will the grade of liver fibrosis and hyperferritinemia as well as T2DM ameliorate by degrees. This modification by treating SAS with CPAP will complicate the clinical data, manifestations and susceptibility to newly developed drugs for NAFLD/NASH patients.

7.6 With or without 'reactive oxygen species (ROS) and Antioxidant dynamics'

A 'two-hit' theory has been postulated to help explain the mechanisms underlying the development of advanced NAFLD. The 'second hit' has yet to be completely described; extensive research has identified several possible mechanisms, including oxidative stress (OS)-induced inflammation with lipid peroxidation, cytokine activation and excess production of reactive oxygen and nitrogen species (ROS/RNS) [124].

The main source of radicals in biological systems is molecular oxygen, which readily accepts electrons, the most important of which being the hydroxyl radical (•OH), the superoxide anion ($O_2^{\bullet -}$) and nitric oxide radical (NO•). These unstable and reactive radicals are natural by-products of the intracellular metabolism and from exogenous substances, which have the ability to react with biological compounds including proteins, FFA and DNA [136, 137]. On the other hand, the main endogenous intracellular sources of ROS are mitochondria, the endoplasmic reticulum (ER) and peroxisomes, superoxide anion radicals ($O_2^{\bullet -}$) are produced because of enzymatic activity, such as with xanthine oxidase (XO) and cytochrome P450 metabolism [107, 138].

In a normal situation, a fine balance exists between prooxidant and antioxidant mechanisms, and OS, which has been long recognised as a key mechanism responsible for liver damage and disease progression in NAFLD, is believed to occur due to an imbalance in favour of prooxidation [139]. Numerous pieces of evidence accumulated over the past decade suggest that mitochondrial dysfunction plays a significant role in steatosis and steatohepatitis. ROS overproduction is induced by mitochondrial dysfunction, and the ensuing increase in the lipid peroxidation and protein oxidation has a detrimental effect on fat homeostasis in the liver. Mitochondria remain the main source of ROS in hepatocytes, although other subcellular organelles have also been shown to participate in the process [140, 141].

As a matter of fact, peroxisomes can oxidise long-chain FFA more rapidly than mitochondria, thereby increasing the cell's capacity to metabolise FFA. However, H_2O_2, which is an end-product of peroxisomal β-oxidation, is converted into the highly reactive OH radical with ease. By promoting toxic accumulation of ROS, which triggers other signalling pathways within the cell, chronic ER stress may also contribute to OS. The relationship between ER stress and OS works both ways because ROS generated through inflammation or damage to organelles (e.g., mitochondria) may also accelerate ER dysfunction [140, 141].

Because of either excessive production of ROS within the hepatocyte or reduced antioxidant defences, oxidative stress occurs and accumulates within the hepatocytes. Most antioxidant enzymes, copper/zinc superoxide dismutase (Cu/Zn SOD) and manganese-superoxide dismutase (MnSOD), which are mainly present in the cytoplasm and mitochondria, promote the reduction of $O_2^{\bullet-}$ to H_2O_2. Another antioxidant enzyme, glutathione peroxidase (GPx), facilitates the subsequent conversion of H_2O_2 to H_2O [137]. In correlation with disease severity, a breakdown in the antioxidant defences plays a significant role in OS associated with NASH, as evidenced by decreased hepatic glutathione (GSH) and diminished SOD, GPx, catalase and glutathione transferase activities [107].

Lipid peroxidation to release more reactive aldehydes is augmented by the resultant increase in mitochondrial ROS, which further damages the mitochondrial DNA (mtDNA) and respiratory chain polypeptides [142].

In summary, mitochondrial dysfunction not only impairs fat homeostasis in the liver but also leads to an overproduction of ROS, which is deliberated to be an important factor in producing lethal hepatocyte injury associated with NAFLD [107].

7.7 With or without 'liver fibrosis and promoting signals'

It is interesting that iron-loading is frequently observed in chronic liver diseases regardless of the aetiology. The Fenton reaction is induced by excessive iron. At the same time, it generates unquenchable amounts of free radicals that cause grave cellular and tissue damage and thereby contribute to fibrosis. In addition, excess iron can induce fibrosis-promoting signals in the parenchymal and non-parenchymal cells, which accelerate disease progression and exacerbate liver pathology. Liver fibrogenesis is the normal process of tissue repair. It is mediated via a complex network of interrelated and regulated signalling interactions between the resident parenchymal cells (hepatocytes), non-parenchymal cells, Kupffer cells, hepatic stellate cells (HSCs), liver sinusoidal endothelial cells, biliary epithelial cells, liver associated lymphocytes and non-resident infiltrating immune cells. HSCs located in the space of Disse between the hepatocytes and liver sinusoids play a pivotal role in liver development and regeneration via fibrogenesis [143].

The fruitless regenerative response perpetuates variable repair-related expansion of immature liver cells, inflammation, vascular remodelling and fibrogenesis, which results in more advanced or severe NASH. By degrees, functional hepatic parenchyma is progressively replaced by scar, and the liver becomes enriched with neoplastic immature hepatocytes; this can account for the increased risk of cirrhosis and liver cancer in patients with severe NASH [144].

The histologic features of NASH indicate the ongoing repair responses to chronic hepatocyte lipotoxicity and vary with the severity of lipotoxicity and success of the wound-healing process. The liver can usually undergo repair and regeneration after acute injury or when chronic injury causes a minor increase in the rate of hepatocyte death. Therefore, there is no progressive replacement of hepatic parenchyma with scar, and the risk for liver cancer remains low in numerous patients with minimal hepatic lipotoxicity and mild NASH [120].

In conclusion, the findings indicate that HSCs, during fibrogenesis in vivo, may not be directly subjected to oxidant stress, and when exposed to various oxidant stressors in vitro, do not turn on the fibrogenic machinery.

7.8 With or without 'amenorrhea or menopause complicated with Mets'.

In menopausal women, oestrogen is one of important hormones for the regulation of glucose metabolism, because it has capacity in exerting a protective effect on pancreatic beta cells and plays an important role in regulating appetite and improving insulin resistance in insulin target organs. It is one of the crucial problems that oestrogen may also play an important role in the progression of NAFLD and NASH. It has been empirically considered that postmenopausal women are at an increased risk of NAFLD and might show metabolic features of insulin resistance. For example, increased total and visceral adiposity in peri- and postmenopausal women is associated with an increased risk of insulin resistance, dyslipidaemia, hypertension, diabetes and cardiovascular disease. Furthermore, postmenopausal women with NAFLD are at an increased risk of portal inflammation, ballooning and fibrosis due to their inability to suppress oxidative stress and fibrosis by lowering their oestrogen levels [145].

It is really recognised that oestrogen replacement therapy has some beneficial effects in patients with liver fibrosis. The risk of NAFLD is greater among postmenopausal women than among premenopausal women [146].

It is possible that the loss of protection conferred by oestrogens', combined with other factors, underlies the increased NAFLD risk in postmenopausal women. NAFLD can easily progress to a more dangerous condition called NASH, which indicates there is both inflammation and liver cell damage, along with fat in the liver [147].

In addition, menopause or amenorrhea actually means 'relative iron overload' for women who develop obesity at the same time. These women have a high risk of deteriorating NAFLD/NASH. In such situations, Laennec as a 'hepcidin inducer' might be a preferable and effective treatment. In my experiences, 13 biopsy-proven NASH cases were extremely sensitive to placenta-derived Laennec treatment. In five cases, second liver biopsy revealed a diminishing liver fibrosis and inflammation, as well as a decrease in iron deposition. In these NASH cases, iron deposition was mainly observed in the Kupffer cells [73, 74, 78].

7.9 With or without 'lipolysis and lipotoxicity'

In discussing the prognosis of liver steatosis, NAFLD does not necessarily lead to NASH because NAFLD is an extremely heterogeneous condition. This heterogeneity exists in part because different types of lipids with different cytotoxic potentials accumulate in the NAFLD, and individuals with NAFLD differ in their ability to defend against lipotoxicity. Differences in these wound-healing responses among individuals determine whether the lipotoxic livers regenerate, leading to stabilisation or resolution of NASH, or develop progressive scarring, cirrhosis and possibly liver cancer.

The perception that the lipotoxic potential of various types of lipids differs can help explain why the outcomes of hepatic steatosis vary as a matter of fact. Interventions that block the accumulation of lipotoxic lipids might, therefore, be used to prevent or treat NASH. Multiplying of fatty acids within the mitochondria could also dissipate the protonmotive force that typically occurs during mitochondrial respiration [148]. This makes mitochondria more vulnerable to other insults that collapse the mitochondrial membrane potential, such as tumour necrosis factor alpha

(TNFα), and could lead to the release of mitochondrial factors that promote apoptosis [149]. Complete cessation of the mitochondrial electron transport and ATP synthesis is caused by extreme depolarisation of mitochondrial membranes, resulting in cellular necrosis [150]. Because damaged mitochondria cannot efficiently metabolise fatty acids, fatty acids accumulate [151], leading to further hepatic lipid accumulation [152], and promoting inflammatory [153] and fibrogenic responses as well as mitogenic responses that could be carcinogenic [154].

Lipotoxicity induces several different types of cellular stresses, including ER stress [154] and impaired autophagy [155]. In addition, it promotes a sterile inflammatory response that can potentiate liver cell injury and death. At the adipocyte level, metabolic dysregulation because of impaired insulin post-receptor signalling leads to excess lipolysis of triglycerides (TGs) and NEFA release into the circulation. At the molecular level, lipotoxicity leads to endoplasmic reticulum (ER) stress, lysosomal dysfunction, inflammasome activation, cell death and activation of inflammatory responses due to lethal and sublethal hepatocellular injury [156].

NASH occurs because lipotoxic hepatocytes release factors that initiate wound-healing responses to replace dying hepatocytes [157]. Wound healing is a complex multi-faceted process that can restore the liver structure and function to a healthy state [158].

7.10 With or without 'the intestinal microbiome and enterohepatic circulation'

While the causal links between the microbiota and NAFLD have not been fully elucidated, disruption in intestinal permeability [159] and bacterial-derived ligands (e.g., LPS) and metabolites (e.g., secondary bile acids, short chain fatty acids) are putative mediators of this association.

It was elucidated recently that the presence of bacterial strain (*Klebsiella pneumoniae*), which produces high levels of endogenous alcohol was associated with NAFLD in a human cohort [160]. Bile acids are synthesised and secreted by hepatocytes and are involved in the absorption of dietary lipids. They are transported back to the liver by enterohepatic circulation and act on the nuclear farnesoid X receptor (FXR), which is also expressed on hepatocytes, thereby affecting glucose [161] and lipid metabolism. Further, the release of FGF after ileal FXR activation is a feedback mechanism that reduces bile acid synthesis, hepatic steatosis and IR [162]. Through their antimicrobial effects, bile acids also modulate the relationship between gut microbiota and chronic liver disease [163] and improve glucose metabolism by activation of G-protein coupled bile acid receptor (GPBAR1) in enterocytes. Therefore, targeting these mechanisms, for example, with an FXR agonist, is an attractive strategy for NAFLD therapy [164]. Gut-derived hormones, such as GLP-1, play a crucial role in controlling nutrient intake, absorption and metabolism and are attractive targets for metabolic disease in general, as well as in the liver [96].

7.11 With or without small amount of alcohol, so-called 'NASH + ASH'

NAFLD and alcohol-related fatty liver disease (AFLD) [165] are already undoubtedly, and will continue to be, leading drivers of progressive liver disease and hepatocellular carcinoma (HCC) worldwide. Severe alcohol abuse leads to accelerated disease progression with higher rates of HCC, liver-related deaths and poor prognosis. In contrast, NAFLD is most frequently related to metabolic dysfunction (MAFLD: metabolic dysfunction-associated fatty liver disease) and is associated with an increased risk of cardiometabolic disease and cancer.

Although the main environmental triggers of fat accumulation differ between AFLD and NAFLD, they are frequently superimposed, and the pathogenesis of inflammation and progressive liver damage share numerous mechanisms [166].

The progression of liver damage is accelerated when, especially at times of acute insults during the natural history of the disease, excess fat and lipotoxicity lead to inflammation, hepatocellular damage and fibrogenesis, in a condition referred to as 'steatohepatitis' (NASH and acute alcohol-related steatohepatitis (ASH)) [167].

Just as all heavy drinkers do not progress to cirrhosis and HCC, nor do all patients with non-alcoholic steatosis progress. However, if NASH patients drink small amounts (EtOH: male <210 g/w, female <140 g/w) of alcohol, in my clinical experience of following more than 200 biopsy-proven NASH patients, the progression of liver fibrosis and deposition of iron at the hepatocytes seem to be more conspicuous compared to those who do not drink any alcohol.

A small amount of alcohol seems to modify and accelerate clinical manifestation and the progression of NASH.

8. How to find a breakthrough for NAFLD/NASH treatment?

As mentioned before, NAFLD/NASH is in general a heterogeneous group of chronic liver diseases characterised by the accumulation of fat in the liver. The heterogeneity and variation of NAFLD/NASH as well as the sensitivity to many kinds of treatment procedures are reflected in a clinical and histologic spectrum, where some patients develop isolated steatosis of the liver, termed non-alcoholic fatty liver, whereas others develop hepatocyte injury, ballooning, inflammation and consequent fibrosis termed as NASH and progress to liver cirrhosis/hepatocellular carcinoma.

Further research is required to determine why progressive scarring develops in only some patients with NASH, define the mechanisms that shift effective regeneration to pathologic scarring [168] and determine how wound-healing responses might be modulated to heal lipotoxicity without scarring [169].

Based on these findings, the risk for NASH is determined by the susceptibility of hepatocytes to toxic lipids and potential for repair of lipotoxic liver damage. Therapies for NASH might, therefore, include those that prevent hepatic lipotoxicity by alleviating systemic metabolic stress [170].

A nascent understanding of this heterogeneity would also suggest that 'combination therapy' might be one of the options for preventing the progression of NASH; however, considering the remarkably wide-ranged heterogeneity of the disease, it may be extremely expensive and sometimes futile. One possible treatment procedure might be the trial with 'bioactive drugs', which have multiple sites of action such as 'antioxidant', 'metabolic regulator' and 'anti-inflammatory effects' at the same time. The sites of action brought about by Laennec on NASH treatment might be so to speak "multicentric" and "covering a wide area" comparing with so called newly developing "monotherapy drugs".

The most important mechanism of Laennec/Porcine might be conducted by the regulation of iron metabolism, which is needed in many kinds of biochemical and biophysical reactions (**Figure 9**). Laennec/Porcine might act on multiple targets, affecting diverse pathological processes and leading to an increased ability to adapt.

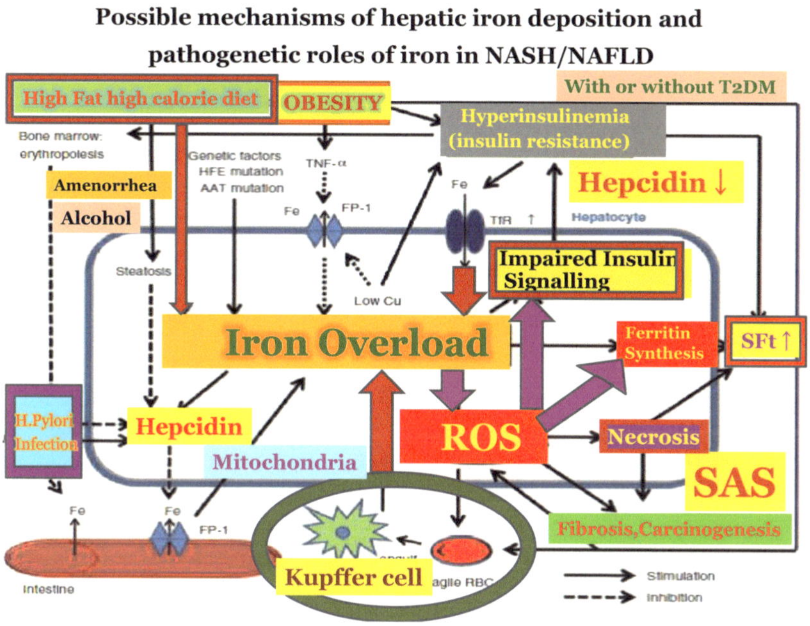

Figure 9.
Possible mechanisms of hepatic iron deposition and pathogenetic roles of iron in NASH/NAFLD. 'Iron reduction therapy' such as phlebotomy or dietary iron restriction may be promising for patients with NASH/NAFLD to reduce insulin resistance as well as serum transaminase activities. Iron is a potent catalyst of oxidative stress and may act synergistically with other promoters of lipid peroxidation by catalysing these reactions. Iron overload can also directly cause lipid peroxidation, and one of the subsequent products, malondialdehyde, has been shown to activate HSCs in vitro, the major source of fibrogenesis in liver injury. Excessive triglyceride accumulation is the most likely first step. The second step may be related to an increase in oxidative stress, which in turn, triggers liver cell necrosis and activation of HSCs, both leading to fibrosis and ultimately to the development of cirrhosis. One of the potential cofactors suspected to enhance this oxidative stress is excessive hepatic iron accumulation (by the courtesy of Ref. [171], partially modified by the author).

This fits seamlessly in the pathophysiologic model of NAFLD/NASH since diverse pathological processes are involved. This concept is really compatible with the site of action induced by Laennec/Porcine. So that, Laennec/Porcine is capable of covering wide range of pathological abnormalities in NAFLD/NASH (**Figures 10** and **11**). If the drug is safe, has no apparent side effects, is cost beneficial (250–300 USD/m), has multiple mechanisms, which will ameliorate NAFLD/NASH spectrum according to the individual pathogenic background, and its pharmacodynamics are clarified, attempts should be made to use such a drug for treating the patients with NAFLD/NASH (**Figures 10** and **11**).

In conclusion, considering numerous factors being involved in the pathogenesis of NAFLD/NASH, one of the most preferable and reliable drugs for the control of these diseases might be the "Bioactives" such as Laennec/Porcine, which have multi-ranged sites of action and the potential to modulate iron metabolism appropriately through the action of "hepcidin inducer".

Further studies should confirm the role of iron overload and the meaning of hyperferritinemia in patients with chronic liver diseases, including NAFLD/NASH. 'Hepcidin inducing therapy' using Laennec/Porcine might be one of the preferable treatment options for controlling wide-ranged NAFLD/NASH along with complicating T2DM (**Figures 10** and **11**).

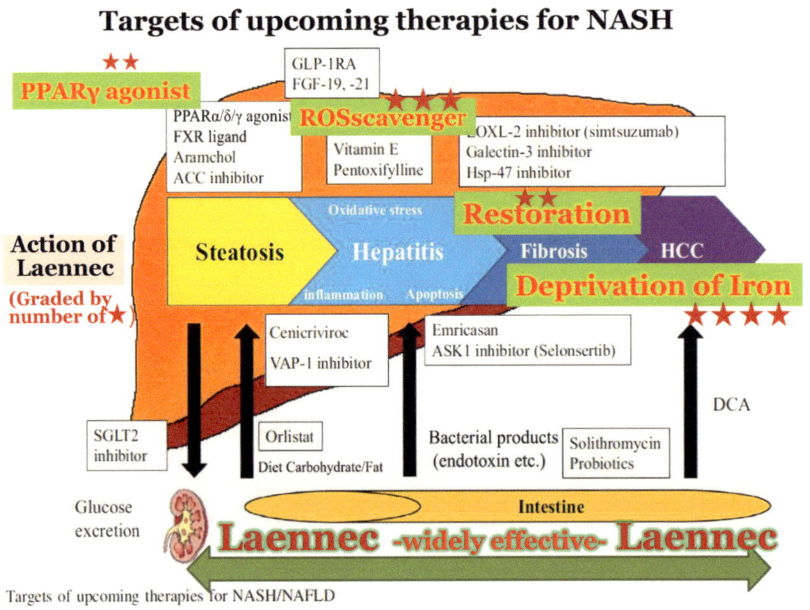

Figure 10.

Targets of upcoming therapies for NASH are shown in this figure. The supposed sites of action of Laennec seem to be widespread compared with those of other newly developed 'single targeted drugs'. The expected sites of action of Laennec are graded ★★—★★★★ tentatively judging from formerly obtained data and clinical observations (by the courtesy of Ref. [172], partially modified by the author).

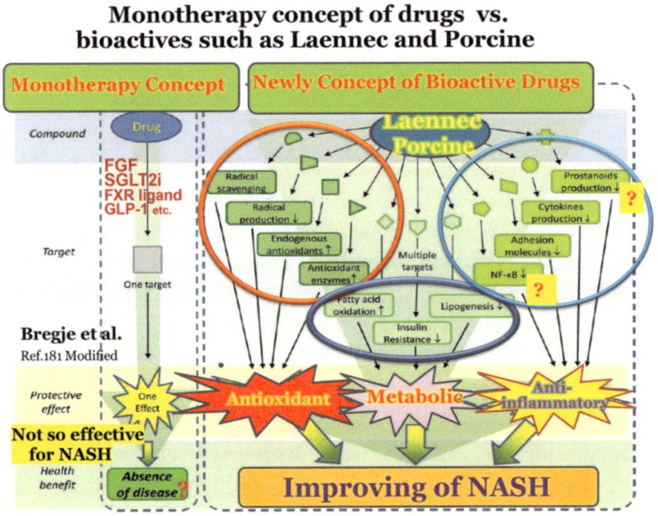

Figure 11.

Traditional concept of drugs vs. the mode of actions (Laennec and Porcine), 'traditional' concept of action of drugs versus the contemporary concept of mode of actions such as Laennec and Porcine. Traditional drugs are developed to act on one target, leading to the absence of disease; however, the target diseases are complicated and consist of many kinds of factors. Laennec and Porcine act on multiple targets, affecting diverse pathological processes and leading to increased ability to adapt. This fits seamlessly in the pathophysiologic model of NAFLD since it involves diverse pathological processes. (Dr. Bregje Van De Wier, Ref. [173], partially modified by the author)

DOI: http://dx.doi.org/10.5772/intechopen.107221

Author details

Yuki Hamada[1] and Eiichi Hirano[2*]

1 Hamada Clinic for Gastroenterology and Hepatology, Sapporo, Japan

2 Laennec Regenerative Medicine Research Center, Japan Bio Products Co., Ltd., Kurume, Japan

*Address all correspondence to: ehirano@placenta-jbp.co.jp

References

[1] Loomba R, Sanyal AJ. The global NAFLD epidemic. Nature Reviews. Gastroenterology & Hepatology. 2013;**10**:686-690

[2] Chalasani N, Younossi Z, et al. The diagnosis and management of nonalcoholic fatty liver disease. Practice guidance from the American Association for the Study of Liver Diseases. Hepatology. 2018;**67**:328-357

[3] Anstee QM, Targher G, Day CP. Progression of NAFLD to diabetes mellitus, cardiovascular disease or cirrhosis. Nature Reviews. Gastroenterology & Hepatology. 2013;**10**:330-344

[4] Charlton MR, Burns JM, et al. Frequency and outcomes of liver transplantation for nonalcoholic steatohepatitis in the United States. Gastroenterology. 2011;**141**:1249-1253

[5] Vernon G, Baranova A, et al. Systematic review: The epidemiology and natural history of non-alcoholic fatty liver disease and non-alcoholic steatohepatitis in adults. Alimentary Pharmacology & Therapeutics. 2011;**34**:274-285

[6] Khan FZ, Perumpail RB, et al. Advances in hepatocellular carcinoma: Nonalcoholic steatohepatitis-related hepatocellular carcinoma. World Journal of Hepatology. 2015;**7**:2155-2161

[7] Lade A, Noon LA, et al. Contributions of metabolic dysregulation and inflammation to nonalcoholic steatohepatitis, hepatic fibrosis, and cancer. Current Opinion in Oncology. 2014;**26**:100-107

[8] Cheung O, Sanyal AJ. Recent advances in nonalcoholic fatty liver disease. Current Opinion in Gastroenterology. 2010;**26**:202-208

[9] Day CP, James OFW. Steatohepatitis: A tale of two "hits"? Gastroenterology. 1998;**114**:842-845

[10] Tilg H, Moschen AR. Evolution of inflammation in nonalcoholic fatty liver disease: The multiple parallel hits hypothesis. Hepatology. 2010;**52**:1836-1846

[11] Harrison SA, Schenker S. Nonalcoholic steatohepatitis: What we know in the new millennium. The American Journal of Gastroenterology. 2002;**97**:2714-2724

[12] Washington K, Wright K, Shyr Y, Hunter EB, Olson S, Raiford DS. Hepatic stellate cell activation in nonalcoholic steatohepatitis and fatty liver. Human Pathology. 2000;**31**:822-828

[13] Ganz T. Molecular control of iron transport. Journal of the American Society of Nephrology. 2007;**18**(2):394-400

[14] Pietrangelo A. Iron in NASH, chronic liver diseases and HCC how much iron is too much? Journal of Hepatology. 2009;**50**(2):249-251

[15] Fargion S et al. Beyond hereditary hemochromatosis: New insights into the relationship between iron overload and chronic liver diseases. Digestive and Liver Disease. 2011;**43**(2):89-95

[16] Ganz T. Hepcidin, a key regulator of iron metabolism and mediator of anemia of infammation. Blood. 2003;**102**(3):783-788

[17] Camaschella C et al. Iron metabolism and iron disorders revisited

in the hepcidin era. Haematologica. 2020;**105**(2):260-272

[18] Valenti L, Moscatiello S, et al. Venesection for non-alcoholic fatty liver disease unresponsive to lifestyle counselling—A propensity score-adjusted observational study. QJM. 2011;**104**:141-149

[19] Fleming RE, Ponka P. Iron overload in human disease. The New England Journal of Medicine. 2012;**366**:348-359

[20] Nascimbeni F, Pais R, Bellentani S, Day CP, Ratziu V, Loria P, et al. From NAFLD in clinical practice to answers from guidelines. Journal of Hepatology. 2013;**59**:859-871

[21] Fujita N, Takei Y. Iron overload in nonalcoholic steatohepatitis. Advances in Clinical Chemistry. 2011;**55**:105-132

[22] Daher R, Lefebvre T. Extrahepatic hepcidin production: The intriguing outcomes of recent years. World Journal of Clinical Cases. 2019;7(15):1926-1936

[23] Valko M, Jomova K, Rhodes CJ, Kuča K, Musílek K. Redox- and non-redox-metal-induced formation of free radicals and their role in human disease. Archives of Toxicology. 2016;**90**:1-37

[24] Muckenthaler MU, Rivella S, Hentze MW, et al. A red carpet for iron metabolism. Cell. 2017;**168**:344

[25] Girelli D, Nemeth E, Swinkels DW. Hepcidin in the diagnosis of iron disorders. Blood. 2016;**127**:2809

[26] Dongiovanni P, Fracanzani AL, Fargion S, Valenti L. Iron in fatty liver and in the metabolic syndrome: A promising therapeutic target. Journal of Hepatology. 2011;**55**:920-932

[27] Nelson JE, Klintworth H, Kowdley KV. Iron metabolism in nonalcoholic fatty liver disease. Current Gastroenterology Reports. 2012;**14**:8-16

[28] Simcox JA, McClain DA. Iron and diabetes risk. Cell Metabolism. 2013;**17**:329-341

[29] Smith BW, Adams LA. Nonalcoholic fatty liver disease and diabetes mellitus: Pathogenesis and treatment. Nature Reviews. Endocrinology. 2011;**7**:456-465

[30] Babitt JL, Lin HY. The molecular pathogenesis of hereditary hemochromatosis. Seminars in Liver Disease. 2011;**31**:280-292

[31] Watt RK. The many faces of the octahedral ferritin protein. Biometals. 2011;**24**:489-500

[32] Larter CZ, Chitturi S, Heydet D, Farrell GC. A fresh look at NASH pathogenesis. Part 1: The metabolic movers. Journal of Gastroenterology and Hepatology. 2010;**25**:672-690

[33] Carmen GY, Víctor SM. Signalling mechanisms regulating lipolysis. Cellular Signalling. 2006;**18**:401-408

[34] Donnelly KL, Smith CI, Schwarzenberg SJ, Jessurun J, Boldt MD, Parks EJ. Sources of fatty acids stored in liver and secreted via lipoproteins in patients with nonalcoholic fatty liver disease. The Journal of Clinical Investigation. 2005;**115**:1343-1351

[35] Samuel VT, Shulman GI. Mechanisms for insulin resistance: Common threads and missing links. Cell. 2012;**148**:852-871

[36] Nelson JE, Wilson L, Brunt EM, Yeh MM, Kleiner DE, UnalpArida A, et al. Relationship between the pattern of hepatic iron deposition and histological severity in nonalcoholic fatty liver disease. Hepatology. 2011;**53**:448-457

[37] Nemeth E, Tuttle MS, Ganz T, et al. Hepcidin regulates cellular iron efflux by binding to ferroportin and

inducing its internalization. Science. 2004;**306**(5704):2090-2093

[38] Barisani D, Pelucchi S, Mariani R, Meneveri R, et al. Hepcidin and iron-related gene expression in subjects with dysmetabolic hepatic iron overload. Journal of Hepatology. 2008;**49**:123-133

[39] Bekri S, Gual P, et al. Increased adipose tissue expression of hepcidin in severe obesity is independent from diabetes and NASH. Gastroenterology. 2006;**131**:788-796

[40] Sumida Y, Nakashima T, Yoh T, et al. Serum thioredoxin elucidates the significance of serum ferritin as a marker of oxidative stress in chronic liver diseases. Liver. 2001;**21**:295-299

[41] Leclercq IA, Farrell GC, Field J, et al. CYP2E1 and CYP4A as microsomal catalysts of lipid peroxides in murine nonalcoholic steatohepatitis. The Journal of Clinical Investigation. 2000;**105**:1067-1075

[42] Ford ES, Cogswell ME. Diabetes and serum ferritin concentration among U.S. adults. Diabetes Care. 1999;**22**:1978-1983

[43] Bugianesi E, Manzini P, Rizzetto M, et al. Relative contribution of iron burden, HFE mutations, and insulin resistance to fibrosis in nonalcoholic fatty liver. Hepatology. 2004;**39**:179-187

[44] Chitturi S, Weltman M, et al. HFE mutations, hepatic iron, and fibrosis: Ethnic-specific association of NASH with C282Y but not with fibrotic severity. Hepatology. 2002;**36**:142-149

[45] Maliken BD, Nelson JE, et al. Hepatic reticuloendothelial system cell iron deposition is associated with increased apoptosis in nonalcoholic fatty liver disease. Hepatology. 2013;**57**:1806-1813

[46] Tan TC, Crawford DH, et al. Excess iron modulates endoplasmic reticulum stress-associated pathways in a mouse model of alcohol and high-fat diet-induced liver injury. Laboratory Investigation. 2013;**93**:1295-1312

[47] Graham RM, Chua AC, Trinder D, et al. Hepatic iron loading in mice increases cholesterol biosynthesis. Hepatology. 2010;**52**:462-471

[48] Jouihan HA, McClain DA, et al. Iron-mediated inhibition of mitochondrial manganese uptake mediates mitochondrial dysfunction in a mouse model of hemochromatosis. Molecular Medicine. 2008;**14**:98-108

[49] Jomova K, Valko M. Advances in metal-induced oxidative stress and human disease. Toxicology. 2011;**283**:65-87

[50] Pinhas-Hamiel, Phillip M, et al. Greater prevalence of iron deficiency in overweight and obese children and adolescents. International Journal of Obesity and Related Metabolic Disorders. 2003;**27**:416-418

[51] Cepeda-Lopez AC, Zimmermann MB, et al. Sharply higher rates of iron deficiency in obese Mexican women and children are predicted by obesity-related inflammation rather than by differences in dietary iron intake. The American Journal of Clinical Nutrition. 2011;**93**:975-983

[52] Azevedo-Martins AK, Tiedge M, et al. Improvement of the mitochondrial antioxidant defense status prevents cytokine-induced nuclear factor-kappaB activation in insulinproducing cells. Diabetes. 2003;**52**:93-101

[53] Montes-Cortes DH, Hicks JJ, et al. Chemical and functional changes of human insulin by in vitro incubation with

blood from diabetic patients in oxidative stress. Metabolism. 2010;**59**:935-942

[54] Ponugoti B, Graves DT, et al. Role of forkhead transcription factors in diabetes-induced oxidative stress. Experimental Diabetes Research. 2012;**93**:9751

[55] Semenza GL. Hypoxia-inducible factors in physiology and medicine. Cell. 2012;**148**:399-408

[56] Shah YM, Gonzalez T, F.J., et al. Intestinal hypoxia-inducible transcription factors are essential for iron absorption following iron deficiency. Cell Metabolism. 2009;**9**:152-164

[57] Fernandez-Real JM, Lopez-Bermejo A, Ricart W. Cross-talk between iron metabolism and diabetes. Diabetes. 2002;**51**:2348-2354

[58] Forouhi NG, Harding AH, Khaw KT, Wareham NJ, et al. Elevated serum ferritin levels predict new-onset type 2 diabetes: Results from the EPIC-Norfolk prospective study. Diabetologia. 2007;**50**:949-956

[59] Borel MJ, Beard JL, Farrell PA. Hepatic glucose production and insulin sensitivity and responsiveness in iron-deficient anemic rats. The American Journal of Physiology. 1993;**264**:E380-E390

[60] Facchini FS. Effect of phlebotomy on plasma glucose and insulin concentrations. Diabetes Care. 1998;**21**:2190

[61] Fernandez-Real JM, Ricart W, et al. Blood letting in high-ferritin type 2 diabetes: Effects on insulin sensitivity and -cell function. Diabetes. 2002;**51**:1000-1004

[62] Shindo T, Yamauchi A, et al. Placental extract ameliorates non-alcoholic steatohepatitis (NASH) by exerting protective effects on endothelial cells. Heliyon. 2017;**3**:e00416. DOI: 10.1016/j.heliyon.2017.e00416

[63] Jung J, Lee, Kim GJ. Placenta extract promote liver regeneration in CCl4-injured liver rat model. International Immunopharmacology. 2011;**11**:976-984

[64] Shimokobe H, Sumida Y, et al. Human placental extract treatment for non-alcoholic steatohepatitis nonresponsive to lifestyle intervention: A pilot study. Hepatology Research. 2014, 2015;**45**(9):1034-1040

[65] Lee KH, Kim TH, Lee, Lee SM. Antiinflammatory and analgesic effects of human placenta extract. Natural Product Research. 2011;**25**:1090-1100

[66] Chen CP, Tsai PS, Huang CJ. Antiinflammation effect of human placental multipotent mesenchymal stromal cells is mediated by prostaglandin E2 via a myeloid differentiation primary response gene 88-dependent pathway. Anesthesiology. 2012;**117**:568-579

[67] Park SY, Phark S. Lee, et al, anti-oxidative and antiinflammatory activities of placental extracts in benzo[a]pyrene-exposed rats. Placenta. 2010;**1**:873-879

[68] Senates E, Yilmaz Y, Ovunc AO, et al. Serum levels of hepcidin in patients with biopsy-proven nonalcoholic fatty liver disease. Metabolic Syndrome and Related Disorders. 2011;**9**:287-290

[69] Dongiovanni P, Lanti C, Valenti L. High fat diet subverts hepatocellular iron uptake determining dysmetabolic iron overload. PLoS One. 2015;**10**:e0116855

[70] Hoki T, Miyanishi K, Tanaka S, et al. Increased duodenal iron absorption through up-regulation of divalent metal

transporter 1 from enhancement of iron regulatory protein 1 activity in patients with nonalcoholic steatohepatitis. Hepatology. 2015;**62**:751-761

[71] Coimbra S, Santos-Silva A, et al. The role of adipocytes in the modulation of iron metabolism in obesity. Obesity Reviews. 2013;**14**:771-779

[72] Siddique A, Nelson JE, Kowdley KV, et al. Iron deficiency in patients with nonalcoholic fatty liver disease is associated with obesity, female gender, and low serum hepcidin. Clinical Gastroenterology and Hepatology. 2014;**12**:1170-1178

[73] Hamada Y, Hirano E. A farewell to phlebotomy—use of placenta-derived drugs Laennec and Porcine for improving hereditary hemochromatosis without phlebotomy: A case report. Journal of Medical Case Reports. 2022;**16**:26. DOI: 10.1186/s13256-021-03230-5

[74] Hamada Y. Laennec derived from human-placenta improves type 2 diabetes complicating with NASH through normalizing iron metabolism by the action of hepcidin. Hepatology International. 2015;**7**(suppl 1):43-48

[75] Hamada Y et al. Laennec can improve type 2 diabetes complicating with NASH through normalizing iron metabolism. Hepatology International. 2016;**10**(S1):S97

[76] Kohgo Y et al. Iron overload and cofactors with special reference to alcohol, hepatitis C virus infection and steatosis/insulin resistance. World Journal of Gastroenterology. 2007;**13**(35):4699-4706

[77] Pietrangelo A. Hepcidin in human iron disorders: Therapeutic implications. Journal of Hepatology. 2011;**54**(1):173-181

[78] Pasricha SR et al. Transfusion suppresses erythropoiesis and increases hepcidin in adult patients with β-thalassemia major: A longitudinal study. Blood. 2013;**122**(1):124-133

[79] Tiedge M et al. Relation between antioxidant enzyme gene expression and antioxidative defense status of insulin-producing cells. Diabetes. 1997;**46**(11):1733-1742

[80] Andrews NC. The iron transporter DMT1. The International Journal of Biochemistry & Cell Biology. 1999;**31**(10):991-994

[81] Kulaksiz H et al. Pancreatic beta-cells express hepcidin, an iron-uptake regulatory peptide. The Journal of Endocrinology. 2008;**197**(2):241-249

[82] Cooksey RC et al. Oxidative stress, beta-cell apoptosis, and decreased insulin secretory capacity in mouse models of hemochromatosis. Endocrinology. 2004;**145**(11):5305-5312

[83] Lunova M et al. Hepcidin knockout mice spontaneously develop chronic pancreatitis owing to cytoplasmic iron overload in acinar cells. The Journal of Pathology. 2017;**241**(1):104-114

[84] Meetei M et al. Study of serum ferritin and HbA1c levels in type 2 diabetes mellitus. Journal of Evidence Based Medicine and Healthcare. 2020;**7**(27):2349-2562

[85] Cooksey RC et al. Dietary iron restriction or iron chelation protects from diabetes and loss of beta-cell function in the obese mouse. American Journal of Physiology. Endocrinology and Metabolism. 2010;**298**(6):E1236-E1243

[86] Tsuchiya H et al. Suppressive effects of retinoids on iron-induced oxidative

stress in the liver. Gastroenterology. 2009;**136**(1):341-350

[87] Senghor A et al. Serum ferritin, iron, TIBC, Hb in male patients with dysglycemia. International Journal of Biological & Medical Research. 2012;**3**(2):1609-1611

[88] Shim JJ. Body iron, serum ferritin, and nonalcoholic fatty liver disease. The Korean Journal of Hepatology. 2012;**18**:105-107

[89] Valenti L, Fracanzani AL, et al. Iron depletion by phlebotomy improves insulin resistance in patients with nonalcoholic fatty liver disease and hyperferritinemia: Evidence from a case-control study. The American Journal of Gastroenterology. 2007;**02**:251-258

[90] Yoneda M, Fujita K, Yoneda K, et al. Serum ferritin is a clinical biomarker in Japanese patients with nonalcoholic steatohepatitis (NASH) independent of HFE gene mutation. Digestive Diseases and Sciences. 2010;**55**:808-814

[91] Beaton MD, Chakrabarti S, Adams PC. Inflammation is not the cause of an elevated serum ferritin in non-alcoholic fatty liver disease. Annals of Hepatology. 2014;**13**:353-356

[92] Valenti L, Bertelli C, et al. Serum ferritin levels are associated with vascular damage in patients with nonalcoholic fatty liver disease. Nutrition, Metabolism, and Cardiovascular Diseases. 2011;**21**:568-575

[93] Canbay A, Feldstein A. Kupffer cell engulfment of apoptotic bodies stimulates death ligand and cytokine expression. Hepatology. 2003;**35**:1188-1198

[94] Kojima Y, Suzuki S. Regulation of pro-inflammatory and anti-inflammatory cytokine responses by kupffer cells in endotoxin-enhanced reperfusion injury after total hepatic ischemia. Transplant International. 2003;**16**:231-240

[95] Younossi ZM, Blissett D, Blissett R, Henry L, Stepanova M, Younossi Y, et al. The economic and clinical burden of nonalcoholic fatty liver disease in the United States and Europe. Hepatology. 2016;**64**:1577-1586

[96] Friedman SL, Neuschwander-Tetri BA, Rinella M, Sanyal AJ. Mechanisms of NAFLD development and therapeutic strategies. Nature Medicine. 2018;**24**:908-922

[97] Hoang SA, Oseini A, Vincent R, et al. Gene expression predicts histological severity and reveals distinct molecular profiles of nonalcoholic fatty liver disease. Scientific Reports. 2019;**9**:12541

[98] Kwok R, Choi KC, Wong GL, et al. Screening diabetic patients for non-alcoholic fatty liver disease with controlled attenuation parameter and liver stiffness measurements: A prospective cohort study. Gut. 2016;**65**:1359-1368

[99] Koehler EM, Plompen EP, Schouten JN, et al. Presence of diabetes mellitus and steatosis is associated with liver stiffness in a general population: The Rotterdam study. Hepatology. 2016;**63**:138-147

[100] Roulot D, Roudot-Thoraval F, Le Clesiau H, Ziol M, Beaugrand M. Concomitant screening for liver fibrosis and steatosis in French type 2 diabetic patients using Fibroscan. Liver International. 2017;**37**:1897-1906

[101] Hamaguchi E, Sakurai M, et al. Histological course of nonalcoholic fatty liver disease in Japanese patients: Tight

glycemic control, rather than weight reduction, ameliorates liver fibrosis. Diabetes Care. 2010;**33**:284-286

[102] Nakahara T, Hyogo H, Yoneda M, et al. Type 2 diabetes mellitus is associated with the fibrosis severity in patients with nonalcoholic fatty liver disease in a large retrospective cohort of Japanese patients. Journal of Gastroenterology. 2014;**49**:1477-1484

[103] Pérez-Carreras M, Del Hoyo P, Martín MA, Martín A, Castellano G, et al. Defective hepatic mitochondrial respiratory chain in patients with nonalcoholic steatohepatitis. Hepatology. 2003;**38**(4):999-1007

[104] Uysal S, Armutcu F, Ikizek M, Yigitoglu MR. Some inflammatory cytokine levels, iron metabolism and oxidan stress markers in subjects with nonalcoholic steatohepatitis. Clinical Biochemistry. 2011;**44**(17-18):1375-1379

[105] Kowdley KV, Belt P, NeuschwanderTetri BA, Nelson JE, et al. Serum ferritin is an independent predictor of histologic severity and advanced fibrosis in patients with nonalcoholic fatty liver disease. Hepatology. 2012;**55**:77-85

[106] Chandok N, Minuk G, et al. Serum ferritin levels do not predict the stage of underlying non-alcoholic fatty liver disease. Journal of Gastrointestinal and Liver Diseases. 2012;**21**:53-58

[107] Rolo AP, Teodoro JS, Palmeira CM. Role of oxidative stress in the pathogenesis of nonalcoholic steatohepatitis. Free Radical Biology & Medicine. 2012;**52**:59-69

[108] Pan M, Fisher EA, et al. Lipid peroxidation and oxidant stress regulate hepatic apolipoprotein B degradation and VLDL production. The Journal of Clinical Investigation. 2004;**113**:1277-1287

[109] Sharp P, Srai SK. Molecular mechanisms involved in intestinal iron absorption. World Journal of Gastroenterology. 2007;**13**:4716-4724

[110] Pigeon C, Loréal O, et al. A new mouse liver-specific gene, encoding a protein homologous to human antimicrobial peptide hepcidin, is overexpressed during iron overload. The Journal of Biological Chemistry. 2001;**276**:7811-7819

[111] Carthew P, Francis JE. Rapid induction of hepatic fibrosis in the gerbil after the parenteral administration of iron-dextran complex. Hepatology. 1991;**13**:534-539

[112] Houglum K, Chojkier M. TGF-beta and collagen-alpha 1 (I) gene expression are increased in hepatic acinar zone 1 of rats with iron overload. The American Journal of Physiology. 1994;**267**:G908-G913

[113] Arezzini B, Lunghi B. Iron overload enhances the development of experimental liver cirrhosis in mice. The International Journal of Biochemistry & Cell Biology. 2003;**35**:486-484

[114] Ramm GA, Crawford DH, Powell LW, Halliday JW. Hepatic stellate cell activation in genetic haemochromatosis. Lobular distribution, effect of increasing hepatic iron and response to phlebotomy. Journal of Hepatology. 1997;**26**:584-592

[115] Gardi C, Arezzini B, et al. Effect of free iron on collagen synthesis, cell proliferation and MMP-2 expression in rat hepatic stellate cells. Biochemical Pharmacology. 2002;**64**:1139-1145

[116] Philippe MA, Ruddell RG, Ramm GA. Role of iron in hepatic

fibrosis: One piece in the puzzle. World Journal of Gastroenterology. 2007;**13**:4746-4754

[117] Aigner E, Weiss G, Datz C. Dysregulation of iron and copper homeostasis in NAFL. World Journal of Hepatology. 2015;7:177-188

[118] Fujita N, Miyachi H, Tanaka H, et al. Iron overload is associated with hepatic oxidative damage to DNA in NASH. Cancer Epidemiology, Biomarkers & Prevention. 2009;**18**:424-432

[119] Siah CW, Ombiga J, Adams LA, et al. Normal iron metabolism and the pathophysiology of iron overload disorders. Clinical Biochemist Reviews. 2006;**27**:5-16

[120] Michelotti GA, Machado MV, Diehl AM. NAFLD, NASH and liver cancer. Nature Reviews. Gastroenterology & Hepatology. 2013;**10**:656-665

[121] Petta S, Craxì A, et al. Non-alcoholic fatty liver disease pathogenesis: The present and the future. Digestive and Liver Disease. 2009;**41**(9):615-625

[122] Armutcu F, Ucar F, et al. Thymosin alpha 1 attenuates lipid peroxidation and improves fructose-induced steatohepatitis in rats. Clinical Biochemistry. 2005;**38**(6):540-547

[123] Diehl AM. Nonalcoholic steatosis and steatohepatitis IV. Nonalcoholic fatty liver disease abnormalities in macrophage function and cytokines. American Journal of Physiology. Gastrointestinal and Liver Physiology. 2002;**282**(1):G1-G5

[124] Seki S, Kitada T, Yamada T, Sakaguchi H, Nakatani K, Wakasa K. In situ detection of lipid peroxidation and oxidative DNA damage in non-alcoholic fatty liver diseases. Journal of Hepatology. 2002;**37**(1):56-62

[125] Senaratna CV, Lodge CJ, et al. Prevalence of obstructive sleep apnea in the general population: A systematic review. Sleep Medicine Reviews. 2017;**34**:70-81

[126] Daltro C, Alves E, et al. Nonalcoholic fatty liver disease associated with obstructive sleep apnea: Just a coincidence? Obesity Surgery. 2010;**20**:1536-1543

[127] Jouët P, Maillard D, et al. Relationship between obstructive sleep apnea and liver abnormalities in morbidly obese patients: A prospective study. Obesity Surgery. 2007;**17**:478-485

[128] James O, Day C. Non-alcoholic steatohepatitis: Another disease of affluence. The Lancet. 1999;**353**:1634-1636

[129] Zamora-Valdés D, Méndez-Sánchez N. Experimental evidence of obstructive sleep apnea syndrome as a second hit accomplice in nonalcoholic steatohepatitis pathogenesis. Annals of Hepatology. 2007;**6**:281-283

[130] Carabelli J, Burgueño AL, Soledad Rosselli M, et al. High fat diet-induced liver steatosis promotes an increase in liver mitochondrial biogenesis in response to hypoxia. Journal of Cellular and Molecular Medicine. 2011;**15**:1329-1338

[131] Byrne TJ, Parish JM, Somers V, et al. Evidence for liver injury in the setting of obstructive sleep apnea. Annals of Hepatology. 2012;**11**:228-231

[132] Acartürk G, Unlü M, Yüksel S, et al. Obstructive sleep apnea, glucose tolerance and liver steatosis in obese women. Journal of Medical Research. 2007;**35**:458-466

[133] Musso G, Cassader M, et al. Obstructive sleep apnea-hypopnea

syndrome and nonalcoholic fatty liver disease: Emerging evidence and mechanisms. Seminars in Liver Disease. 2012;**32**:49-64

[134] Rosmorduc O, Housset C. Hypoxia: A link between fibrogenesis, angiogenesis, and carcinogenesis in liver disease. Seminars in Liver Disease. 2010;**30**:258-270

[135] Zamora-Valdés D, Méndez-Sánchez N. Experimental evidence of obstructive sleep apnea syndrome as a second hit acomplice in nonalcoholic steatohepatitis pathogenesis. Annals of Hepatology. 2007;**6**:281-283

[136] Nomura K, Yamanouchi T. The role of fructose-enriched diets in mechanisms of nonalcoholic fatty liver disease. The Journal of Nutritional Biochemistry. 2012;**23**(3):203-208

[137] Gutteridge JM, Halliwell B. Free radicals and antioxidants in the year 2000. A historical look to the future. Annals of the New York Academy of Sciences;**2000**(899):136-147

[138] Robertson G, Leclercq I, Farrell GC. Nonalcoholic steatosis and steatohepatitis. II. Cytochrome P-450 enzymes and oxidative stress. American Journal of Physiology. Gastrointestinal and Liver Physiology. 2001;**281**(5):G1135-G1139

[139] Begriche K, Igoudjil A, Pessayre D, Fromenty B. Mitochondrial dysfunction in NASH: Causes, consequences and possible means to prevent it. Mitochondrion 2006;6(1):1-28.

[140] Bonekamp NA, Völkl A, Fahimi HD, Schrader M. Reactive oxygen species and peroxisomes: Struggling for balance. Biofactors. 2009;**35**(4):346-355

[141] Cullinan SB, Diehl JA. Coordination of ER and oxidative stress signaling: The PERK/Nrf2 signaling pathway. International Journal of Biochemistry & Cell Biology. 2006;**38**(3):317-332

[142] Sanyal AJ, Campbell-Sargent C, Contos MJ, Sterling RK, et al. Nonalcoholic steatohepatitis: Association of insulin resistance and mitochondrial abnormalities. Gastroenterology. 2001;**120**(5):1183-1192

[143] Lee UE, Friedman SL. Mechanisms of hepatic fibrogenesis. Best Practice & Research. Clinical Gastroenterology. 2011;**25**:195-206

[144] Richardson MM, Jonsson JR, Powell EE, et al. Progressive fibrosis in NASH: Association with altered regeneration and a ductular reaction. Gastroenterology. 2007;**133**:80-90

[145] Suzuki A, Abdelmalek MF. Nonalcoholic fatty liver disease in women. Womens Health (Lond). 2009;**5**:191-203

[146] Pang H et al. Gender and menopause impact severity of fibrosis among patients with nonalcoholic steatohepatitis. Hepatology. 2014;**59**:1406-1414

[147] Kawanaka M, Nishino K. Progression from nonalcoholic fatty liver to nonalcoholic steatohepatitis cirrhosis confirmed by liver histology after 14 years. Internal Medicine. 2021;**60**:1397-1401

[148] Chavin KD, Yang S, Lin HZ, et al. Obesity induces expression of uncoupling protein-2 in hepatocytes and promotes liver ATP depletion. The Journal of Biological Chemistry. 1999;**274**:5692-5700

[149] Cortez-Pinto H, Chatham J, Chacko VP, et al. Alterations in liver ATP homeostasis in human NASH: A pilot study. Journal of the American Medical Association. 1999;**282**:1659-1664

[150] Yang Y, Jiang G, Zhang P, et al. Programmed cell death and its role in inflammation. Military Medical Research. 2015;**2**:12

[151] Koliaki C, Szendroedi J, Kaul K, et al. Adaptation of hepatic mitochondrial function in humans with NAFL is lost in steatohepatitis. Cell Metabolism. 2015;**21**:739-746

[152] Guo S. Insulin signaling, resistance, and the metabolic syndrome: Insights from mouse models into disease mechanisms. The Journal of Endocrinology. 2014;**220**:T1-T23

[153] Miao H, Zhang Y, Lu Z, et al. FOXO1 involvement in insulin resistance-related pro-inflammatory cytokine production in hepatocytes. Inflammation Research. 2012;**61**:349-358

[154] Ashraf NU, Sheikh TA. Endoplasmic reticulum stress and oxidative stress in the pathogenesis of NAFLD. Free Radical Research. 2015;**49**:1405-1418

[155] Amir M, Czaja MJ. Autophagy in NASH. Expert Review of Gastroenterology & Hepatology. 2011;**5**:159-166

[156] Ibrahim SH, Hirsova P, Gores GJ. Non-alcoholic steatohepatitis pathogenesis: Sublethal hepatocyte injury as a driver of liver inflammation. Gut. 2018;**67**:963-972

[157] Angulo P, Machado MV, Diehl AM. Fibrosis in NAFLD: Mechanisms and clinical implications. Seminars in Liver Disease. 2015;**35**:132-145

[158] Machado MV, Diehl AM. Liver renewal: Detecting misrepair and optimizing regeneration. Mayo Clinic Proceedings. 2014;**89**:120-130

[159] Luther J, Garber JJ, Jindal R, et al. Hepatic injury in nonalcoholic steatohepatitis contributes to altered intestinal permeability. Cellular and Molecular Gastroenterology and Hepatology. 2015;**1**:222-232

[160] Yuan J, Chen C, Cui J, Lu J, Yan C, Wei X, et al. Fatty liver disease caused by high-alcohol-producing Klebsiella pneumoniae. Cell Metabolism. 2019;**30**:675-688.e677

[161] Zhang Y, Lee FY, Barrera G, Lee H, Vales C, Gonzalez FJ, et al. Activation of the nuclear receptor FXR improves hyperglycemia and hyperlipidemia in diabetic mice. Proceedings of the National Academy of Sciences of the United States of America. 2006;**103**:1006-1011

[162] Alvarez-Sola G, Uriarte I, Latasa MU, Fernandez-Barrena MG, Urtasun R, Elizalde M, et al. Fibroblast growth factor 15/19 (FGF15/19) protects from diet-induced hepatic steatosis: Development of an FGF19-based chimeric molecule to promote fatty liver regeneration. Gut. 2017;**66**:1818-1828

[163] Parseus A, Sommer N, Sommer F, Caesar R, Molinaro A, Stahlman M, et al. Microbiota-induced obesity requires farnesoid X receptor. Gut. 2017;**66**:429-437

[164] van Nierop FS, Scheltema MJ, Eggink HM, Pols TW, Sonne DP, Knop FK, et al. Clinical relevance of the bile acid receptor TGR5 in metabolism. The Lancet Diabetes and Endocrinology. 2017;**5**:224-233

[165] Eslam M, Sanyal AJ, George J, International Consensus P. MAFLD: A consensus-driven proposed nomenclature for metabolic associated fatty liver disease. Gastroenterology. 2020;**158**:1999-2014

[166] Valenti L, Fracanzani AL, Fargion S. The immunopathogenesis of alcoholic

and nonalcoholic steatohepatitis: Two triggers for one disease? Seminars in Immunopathology. 2009;**31**:359-369

[167] Pelusi S, Cespiati A, Rosso C, et al. Prevalence and risk factors of significant fibrosis in patients with nonalcoholic fatty liver without steatohepatitis. Clinical Gastroenterology and Hepatology. 2019;**17**:2310-2319

[168] Mogler C, Wieland M, Konig C, et al. Hepatic stellate cell-expressed endosialin balances fibrogenesis and hepatocyte proliferation during liver damage. EMBO Molecular Medicine. 2015;**7**:332-338

[169] Ding BS, Cao Z, Lis R, et al. Divergent angiocrine signals from vascular niche balance liver regeneration and fibrosis. Nature. 2014;**505**:97-102

[170] Pritchard MT, McCracken JM. Identifying novel targets for treatment of liver fibrosis: What can we learn from injured tissues which heal without a scar? Current Drug Targets. 2015;**16**:1332-1346

[171] Sumida Y, Okanoue T, et al. Role of hepatic iron in non-alcoholic steatohepatitis. Hepatology Research. 2009;**39**:213-2221

[172] Sumida Y, Yoneda M. Current and future pharmacological therapies for NAFLD/NASH. Journal of Gastroenterology. 2018;**53**:362-376

[173] Van De Wier B, Koek GH, et al. The potential of flavonoids in the treatment of non-alcoholic fatty liver disease. Critical Reviews in Food Science and Nutrition. 2017;**57**(4):834-855

Chapter 6

Therapeutic Approach to NAFLD-NASH

Georgios Sfikas and Ioannis Valsamidis

Abstract

Nonalcoholic fatty liver disease (NAFLD) and its progressive form nonalcoholic steatohepatitis (NASH) are the hepatic expression of metabolic syndrome and may lead to serious injury to the liver resulting in cirrhosis and hepatocellular carcinoma (HCC). Despite its seriousness, there is no definite treatment to address this life-threatening condition. Weight loss and exercise remain the cornerstone of the therapeutic treatment but also an array of medications can be used with varying degrees on liver inflammation and cirrhosis. There is also an increased risk of cardiovascular events connected to NAFLD/NASH, which should also be addressed. Statins have been shown to reduce the lipid and the inflammatory burden of the liver as well as decrease the cardiovascular risk. Aspirin also has a beneficial effect due to its anti-inflammatory properties as well as Vitamin E in certain cases. The medications (metformin, pioglitazone, GLP-1 agonists, SGLT2 inhibitors) that interfere in glucose metabolism and the activity of insulin seem to play a vital role in the metabolism of glucose and lipids and subsequent amelioration of liver function tests and the inhibition of inflammation. The aim of this review is to highlight the efficacy of current therapeutic strategies and explore the variety of the emerging new agents which target newly discovered pathways associated with the pathogenesis of NAFLD/NASH with promising results.

Keywords: nonalcoholic fatty liver disease NAFLD, nonalcoholic steatohepatitis-NASH, metabolic syndrome, obesity, statins, diabetes mellitus

1. Introduction

Nonalcoholic fatty liver disease/nonalcoholic steatohepatitis (NAFLD/NASH) describes a group of diseases that are characterized by hepatic steatosis without the excessive intake of alcohol. NAFLD/NASH may involve cirrhosis and/or hepatocellular carcinoma (HCC). NAFLD may be differentiated from the more benign state of the nonalcoholic liver to nonalcoholic steatohepatitis (NASH), which is the most serious manifestation of the disease. In the first case, hepatic steatosis presents without indication of inflammation, while in NASH hepatic steatosis is connected to lobular inflammation and apoptosis that may lead to fibrosis and cirrhosis [1] (**Figure 1**). Therapeutic management is divided into two kinds of measures: Lifestyle intervention and pharmacological/surgical treatment.

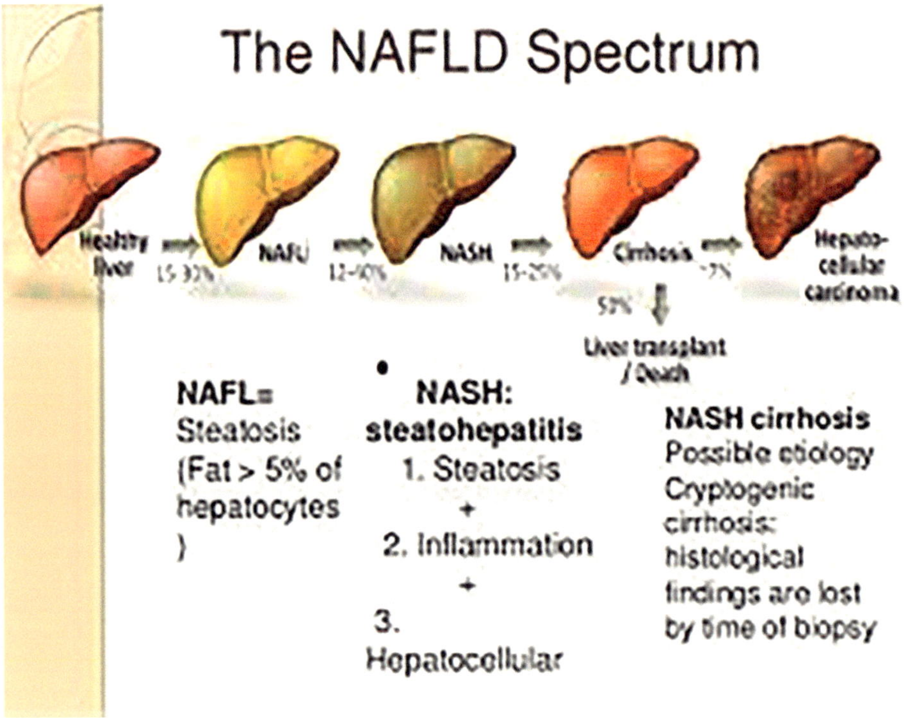

Figure 1.
NAFLD-NASH staging and progression.

2. Lifestyle intervention

2.1 Alcohol abstinence

Patients with NAFLD/NASH are suggested to avoid the use of alcohol and especially to avoid the abuse of it, e.g. fourteen drinks per week or over four drinks per day for male and over seven drinks per week or over three per day for female. The use of alcohol is connected to the progression of the disease [2].

2.2 Regulation of cardiometabolic risk factors

Patients with NAFLD/NASH have an increased risk of cardiovascular disease and they often have multiple risk factors (hypertension, diabetes, dyslipidemia, smoking) (**Figure 2**). The regulation and treatment of these factors have an ameliorating effect on the disease progression and reduce the overall risk of cardiovascular disease [3].

2.3 Physical activity

For people with NAFLD/NASH, exercise is necessary since it regulates metabolism. These people frequently have a tendency towards obesity and metabolic syndrome, whether or not they also have type 2 diabetes. Additionally, they prompt sedentary lifestyles, which accelerates development [4]. According to reports, increasing daily exercise decreases obesity while increasing the metabolism of fatty

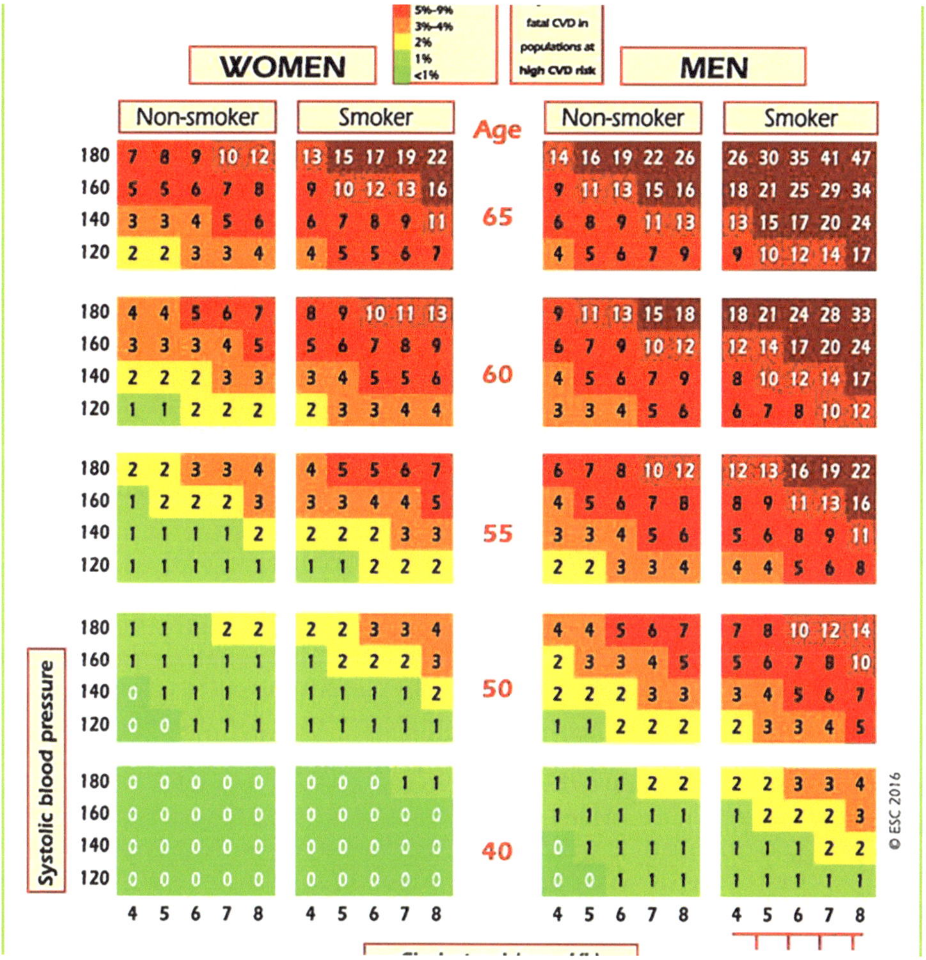

Figure 2.
Score chart: 10-Year risk of fatal cardiovascular disease (CVD).

acids and glucose. Exercise decreases hepatic fat content, as well as adipose tissue and plasma-free fatty acids, which form the pathophysiologic basis for these alterations. It has been demonstrated that activities with higher intensity and longer duration have a more significant impact on cardiometabolic morbidity and mortality as well as greater benefits for NASH and liver fibrosis [5].

2.4 Loss of weight/diet

The loss of weight is the main treatment for most patients with NAFLD/NASH. It is suggested for all patients that are overweight (BMI > 25 kg/m2) or obese (BMI > 30 kg/m2), because weight loss can lead to amelioration of liver function tests, histologic findings, and insulin resistance. It mainly consists of the restriction of intake calories through the decrease of the metabolism of carbohydrates **Table 1.** This reduces the glycemic load, and improves the pancreatic b-cell insulin secretion, it increases HDL-C and further decreases serum triglycerides and glucose [6]. The patients are consulted to lose 5 to 7% of the initial body weight with a rate of 0.5 to 1 kg per week. For patients with NASH (suspected or proven by biopsy), the target of

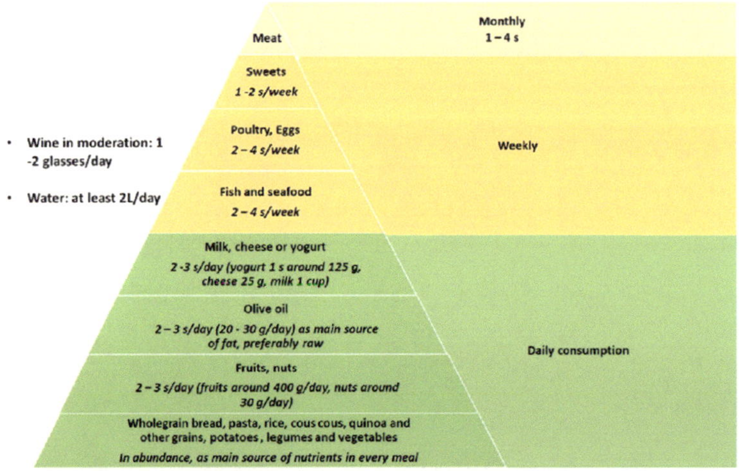

Table 1.
Indicative diet for weight loss in NAFLD/NASH.

weight loss is even higher (7 to 10% of the initial body weight). For some patients, an even greater body loss may be required. If the values of ALT are not normalized, after the achievement of the above-mentioned targets, they are advised to lose even more weight. It has been shown from several studies that at least 5% of the initial body weight is required for the improvement of the hepatic steatosis [7]. In a meta-analysis of eight studies, which include 373 patients, the loss of equal or more to 5% of body weight resulted in the improvement of hepatic steatosis, while the loss of at least 5% of body weight was correlated with a further amelioration of NAFLD/NASH [8]. The above changes need at least a timeline of 6 months to be implemented and reveal significant results.

2.5 Bariatric surgery

Bariatric surgery is an option in patients unresponsive to lifestyle changes and pharmacotherapy. It is currently recommended for patients with BMI > 40 kg/m2 and no comorbidities, or in patients with BMI > 35 kg/m2 and serious comorbidities (T2DM, Hypertension, NAFLD/NASH). A review of 29 studies of patients that underwent bariatric surgery showed a significant improvement in liver function tests and a meta-analysis reported a decrease in steatosis, inflammation, and fibrosis [9, 10].

2.6 Immunization

Patients who do not have serologic verification of immunity should receive the hepatitis A and B vaccines. Pneumococcal vaccination and common immunizations offered to the public are additional vaccines for those with chronic liver disease.

3. Pharmacological treatment

Various pharmacological treatments had been studied for the management of patients with NAFLD/NASH (**Figure 3**). Most of these studies were very short and

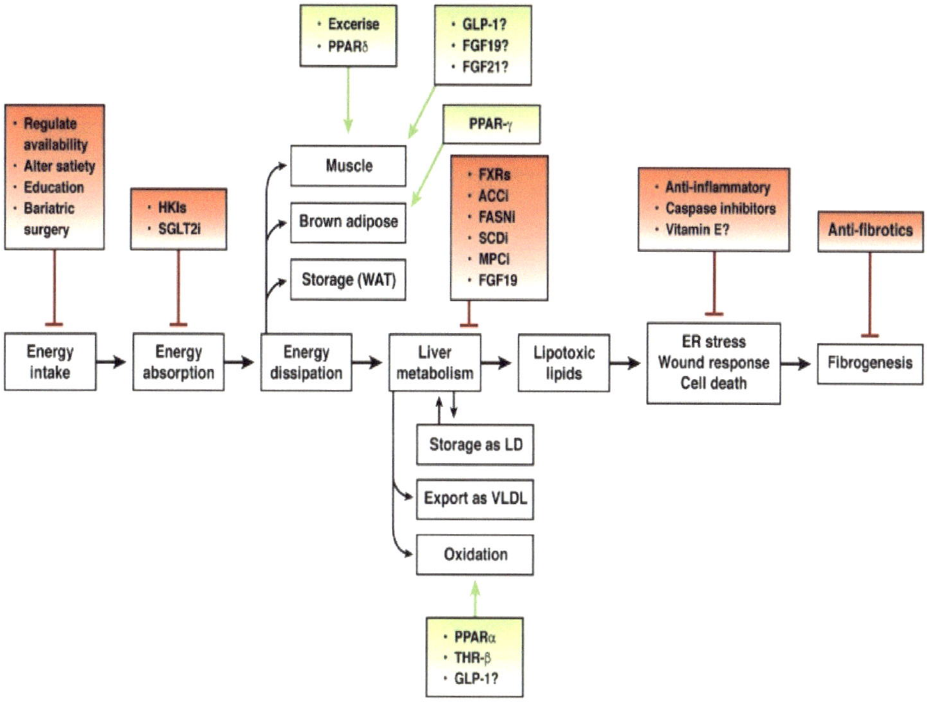

Figure 3.
Pathways in metabolism where pharmaceutical interventions are made.

could not identify a target with important clinical result for the patients (e.g., non-compensated liver cirrhosis), instead referring to certain objective findings, e.g., levels of aminotransferases or histologic findings, often with conflicting results.

3.1 Vitamin E

800 IU of vitamin E per day is typically advised for patients with biopsy-proven NASH and grade of fibrosis equivalent to or more than 2, who do not have diabetes mellitus. According to certain research, vitamin E helps these patients' steatosis. Nevertheless, there are a variety of data and safety issues when vitamin E doses are administered, so potential risks and benefits of treatment with vitamin E should be explored and the decision to use vitamin E should be made on an individual basis [11]. The American Society for the study of liver diseases advises against the use of vitamin E in individuals with compensated liver cirrhosis and DM although studies that demonstrated the benefits of vitamin E treatment did include these patients. The use of vitamin E is supported by some but not all randomized research; however, inconsistent results may be attributed to variations in these studies' design. A meta-analysis of five of these studies could not find histologic benefits with vitamin E, but there was significant heterogeneity among those studies concerning the synthesis of vitamin E that was used, the patient population, the study duration and lifestyle changes. Nevertheless, the biggest of these studies (pioglitazone vs. vitamin E vs. placebo for the treatment of non-diabetic patients with NASH-PIVENS) showed improvements with the use of vitamin E. The study included the randomization of 247 adults with NASH without DM, who received pioglitazone (30 mg per day), Vitamin E (800 IU per day)

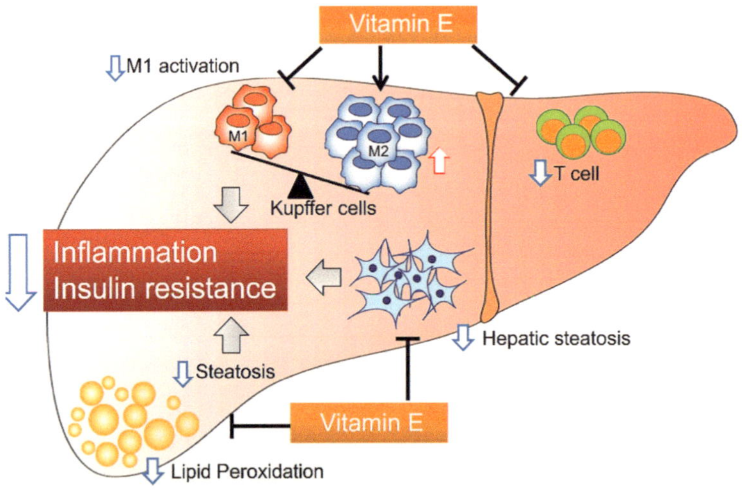

Figure 4.
Action of Vitamin E in NAFLD/NASH.

or placebo for 96 weeks. Patients who were treated with vitamin E, had a higher possibility to have an improvement in the FIB-4 score versus the ones who received placebo (43% vs. 19%) [12]. A meta-analysis of this study showed that the improvement in ALT was more frequent in patients who received vitamin E versus placebo (48% vs. 16%). This is consistent with observational studies that showed improvements in the levels of aminotransferases in patients with NASH that received Vitamin E [13]. This benefit is possibly related to the antioxidative qualities of vitamin E (**Figure 4**). The very high doses of vitamin E (>400 IU per day) have been co-related in conflicting results with the increase in mortality from other comorbidities. So, a very careful approach and individualization is advised. The use of vitamin E should be avoided in male patients with personal or familiar history of prostate cancer [14, 15].

3.2 Aspirin

There is some evidence that patients with NAFLD may benefit from taking aspirin daily. When 361 individuals with biopsy-proven NAFLD were recruited for a prospective cohort trial, those receiving daily aspirin treatment had a lower risk of developing NASH and fibrosis than those who did not get daily aspirin treatment [14]. Additionally, in a 3692-person trial, daily aspirin users were less likely to develop advanced fibrosis than non-users among 317 patients who did not have fibrosis at the time of recruitment. These results are very encouraging, and further research may provide evidence supporting aspirin's hepatoprotective properties [16].

3.3 Statins

The use of statins (HMG-CoA inhibitors) has shown in various studies to improve biochemical and histologic findings in NAFLD/NASH and slow down the progress of fibrosis. These results are attributed to the decrease of the levels of cholesterol and triglycerides, achieved by using statins, as well as their anti-inflammatory properties (**Figure 5**). Moreover, they decrease the cardiovascular risk associated with fatty liver disease [16].

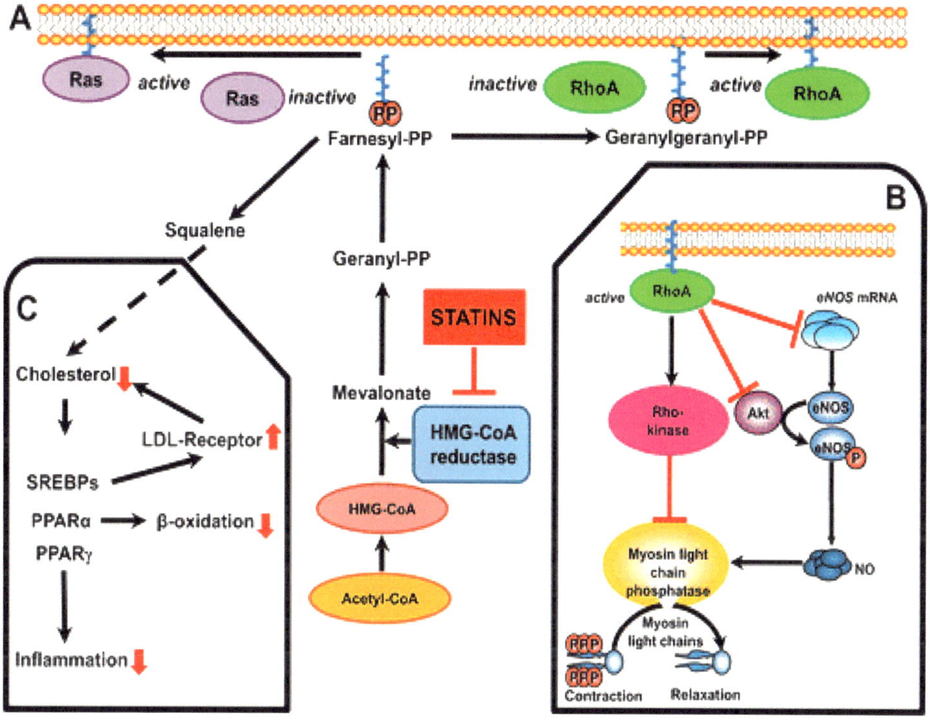

Figure 5.
Pathway of lipid metabolism and statin action in NAFLD/NASH.

Several data, demonstrating the beneficial effect of statins come from the post-hoc analysis of three perspectives, controlled survival studies. The post-hoc analysis of Greek Atorvastatin and Coronary Heart Disease Evaluation (GREACE), included 1600 patients, with coronary heart disease (CHD) and a mean observation time of 3 years. This analysis included 437 patients with NAFLD/NASH. Atorvastatin lowered the levels of serum aminotransferases, normalized the ultrasound imaging of the liver, and decreased cardiovascular events by 64 percent compared to the participants with NAFLD/NASH that did not take statins [17]. Three years later, the researchers of Incremental Decrease in End Points Through Aggressive Lipid Lowering (IDEAL) concluded their post-hoc analysis. IDEAL was carried out in four Scandinavian countries and included 8864 patients with cardiovascular disease, of whom 7782 (87.8%) had normal levels of aminotransferases and 1081 (12.2%) elevated levels of ALT, possibly due to NAFLD/NASH. In the patients with elevated ALT, a dose of atorvastatin 80 mg per day, normalized those levels within safety compared to simvastatin 20–40 mg per day. The most important fact was that the patients who received atorvastatin 80 mg per day, suffered half the number of cardiovascular events, strokes and acute coronary events as those who were treated with simvastatin [18]. This shows that the clinical benefit of the treatment with a statin in NAFLD/NASH is a composite special effect and not the result of a class effect of a category of drugs. There was a post-hoc analysis of primary prevention of a multicenter prospective randomized controlled study: Assessing the treatment effect in Metabolic Syndrome Without Perceptible diabetes (ATTEMPT), that included 1123 patients with a mean observation of 4 years that had similar clinical and biochemical benefits with a higher dose of atorvastatin (30 mg per day) in 326 patients who had moderately elevated levels of hepatic enzymes and ultrasonographic findings of NAFLD. In all the above studies, the patients were included only if the level of aminotransferases were less than three times higher than upper normal levels [19, 20].

Due to the fact that there was no proof of the benefit of the statins in NAFLD/NASH based on liver biopsy, a pilot study was conducted on 20 subjects to evaluate the effect of 10 mg per day of rosuvastatin in biopsy-proven NASH. A year later, 19 of 20 patients, showed a total remission of NASH in new biopsy findings with subsequent normalization of liver enzyme and ultrasonographic findings. Another study from Italy with 107 patients with biopsy-proven NASH showed benefits from statin therapy, as well as a larger study with participants from Italy and France.

In a study performed on 5400 military personnel in Northern Greece, the NASH and FIB-4 scores were used to identify the ones that had NASH and NAFLD/NASH. Their final number was 613 (541 males and 72 females). These subjects were also confirmed to have NAFLD by ultrasonographic findings. They were subsequently divided into four categories: a control group, a group that received rosuvastatin, a group that received atorvastatin and a group that received pitavastatin. The dose of the statins was treated according to individualized LDL-C goals. The results of this study showed a clear benefit in all statin groups compared to the control group, after one year of treatment, which was manifested in the improvement of NASH and FIB-4 scores as well as of the levels of aminotransferases. It should be stressed that the beneficial results of the use of statins were equally important to the subjects without metabolic syndrome, compared to the ones with metabolic syndrome, proving that the use of statins may have a crucial effect on the management of patients with a genetic disposition to present with NAFLD/NASH, independently of the presence of metabolic syndrome [20].

3.4 Ω3-Fatty acids

Studies have suggested that people with NAFLD can benefit from the usage of 3-fatty acids. Treatment with 3-Fatty acids was observed to ameliorate hepatic steatosis as well as the levels of AST in a meta-analysis of nine studies involving 355 individuals. Additionally, there was a tendency for the levels of ALT to rise. Only hepatic steatosis continued to improve with therapy with omega-3 fatty acids when the analysis was limited to randomized trials [21, 22].

3.5 Anti-diabetic drugs

Anti-diabetic medications have been shown to improve outcomes in NAFLD/NASH and consequent liver fibrosis, even without an established diagnosis of diabetes mellitus. This is to a different degree due to their mechanism of modification of the metabolic syndrome (**Figure 6**), the cellular sensitization of insulin, and the effect of insulin itself on tissues.

3.6 Metformin

The principal treatment for diabetes mellitus type 2 is metformin, which is still recommended in all guidelines unless it is contraindicated. It is the primary cellular insulin sensitizer, interfering with insulin resistance, the primary pathophysiologic mechanism of type 2 diabetes [23]. Inhibiting hepatic gluconeogenesis, a supplementary method to promote normal serum glycemia is another effect of it (**Figure 7**). Hypertriglyceridemia is also improved by bringing glucose levels back to normal. Metformin uses improved

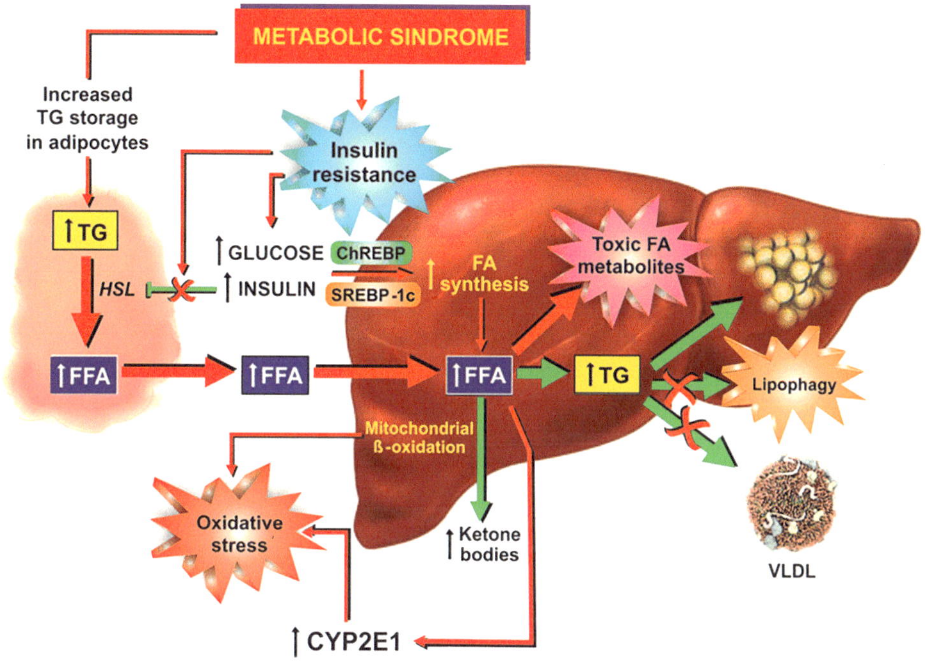

Figure 6.
Pathogenesis of metabolic syndrome.

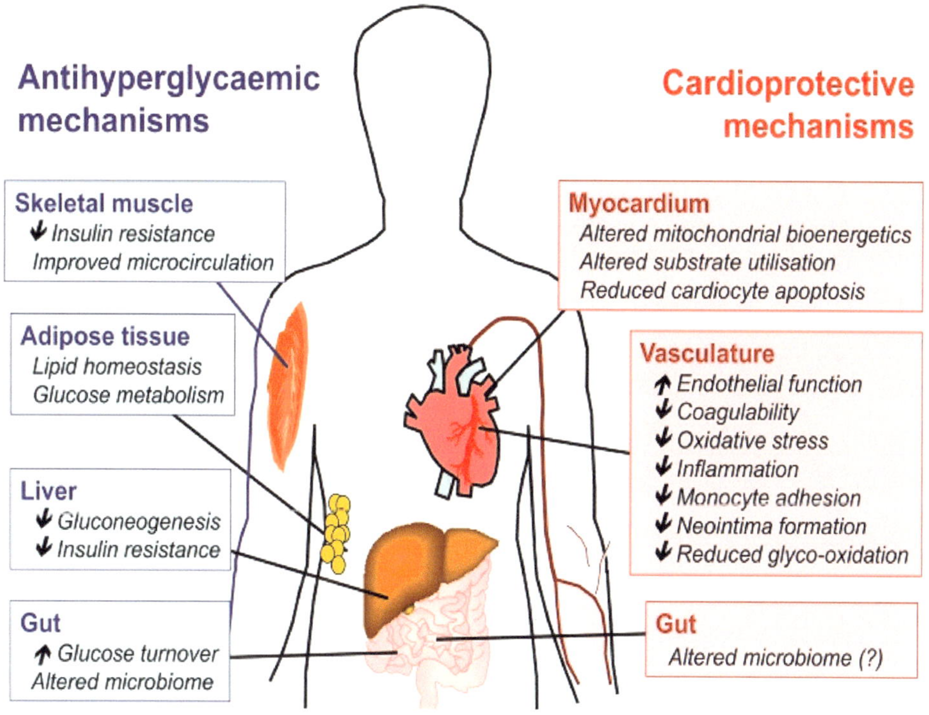

Figure 7.
Action of metformin in multiple sites.

liver ultrasound imaging and the levels of aminotransferases, particularly ALT, according to a meta-analysis of 13 prospective trials, but it did not significantly enhance all patients' histologic findings. Larger studies must be conducted and for a longer period because the number of patients included in these studies was relatively small and they were followed up for a brief period of time (in most cases 6–12 months). This will allow for a better evaluation of the effectiveness of metformin on NAFLD/NASH [24].

3.7 Peroxisome Proliferator-Activated Receptors (PPAR)

The only medication in this class that is currently in use is pioglitazone. It is regarded as an activator of the PPAR nuclear receptor of the PPARγ subgroup, which is mostly expressed in adipose tissue and associated with the reduction of inflammation, adipocyte differentiation, and lipid and glucose metabolism (**Figure 8**). Pioglitazone possibly increases peripheral insulin sensitivity by inducing the release of adipokines, promoting the storage of triglycerides in adipose tissue, and boosting insulin's inhibitory effect on lipolysis. These have the effect of decreasing plasma levels of free fatty acids and causing the liver to reabsorb lipids [25]. Throughout these pathways, it enhances hepatic and peripheral insulin sensitivity and influences the pathophysiology and development of NASH in a beneficial way [13, 26]. The PPARγ sensitizers were reported to improve the hepatic histologic findings of ballooning,

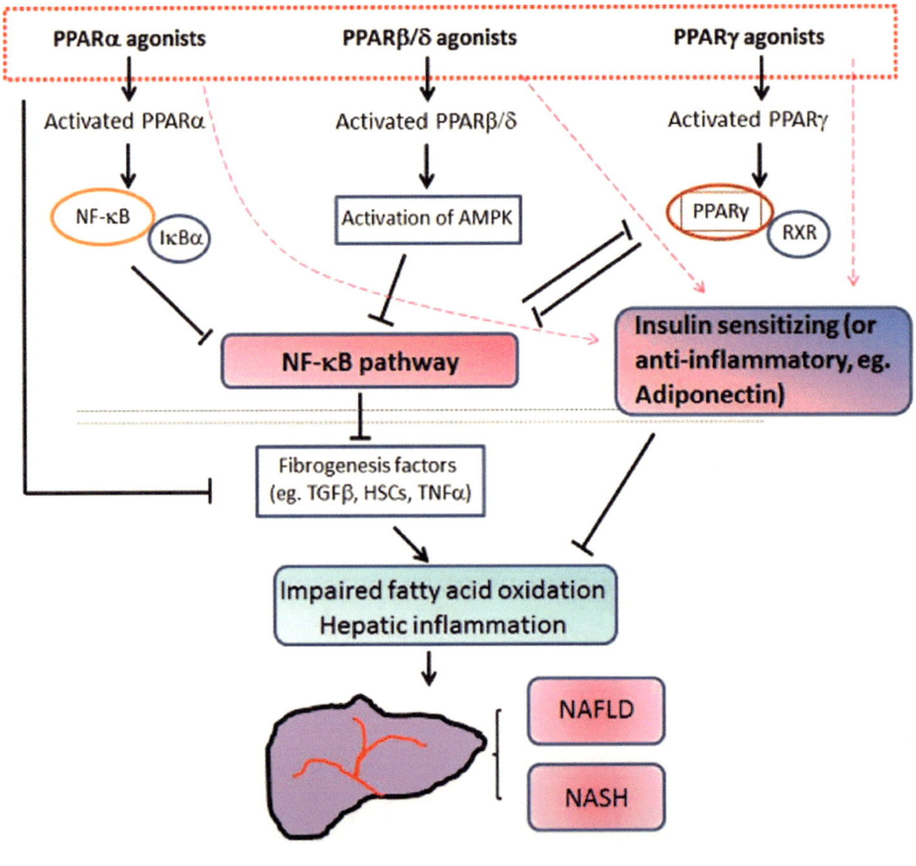

Figure 8.
Action of PPAR sensitizers in NAFLD/NASH.

lobular inflammation, and steatosis in a meta-analysis that compared the use of Thiazolidinediones to placebo in 334 individuals, but no significant improvement of fibrosis was detected. The favorable benefits were reversed following drug termination, which is proof that a prolonged course of treatment is necessary to provide a substantial benefit [26, 27].

Apart from PPARγ agonists, there also are other members of the drug family (PPARα and PPARδ) agonists which are expressed mostly in oxidative tissues and are deeply involved in mitochondrial biogenesis and metabolism, fatty acid oxidation, ketogenesis, and fatty acid uptake-triglyceride metabolism. Elafribranor, a dual PPARα—PPARδ agonist, has been proven in animal models to enhance lipid and insulin metabolism and lessen hepatic inflammation and fibrosis. In animal models, the drug Lanifribranor has demonstrated improved glucose metabolism and decreased steatosis. Saroglitazar, a dual PPARα/γ agonist, also increased insulin sensitivity in people with type 2 diabetes. It also decreased hepatic steatosis and inflammation while preventing fibrosis in animal models. All of these agents are tested in ongoing trials [28–30].

3.8 GLP-1 agonists and DPP-4 inhibitors

GLP-1 is an endogenous hormone of the intestine which acts through the G-protein coupled GLP-1 receptor (GLPR). This directly stimulates the production and release of insulin while simultaneously inhibiting glucagon secretion and reducing food intake. The half-life of GLP-1 in the plasma circulation is only 1–2 minutes, due to the action of dipeptidyl peptidase (DDP-4) which inactivates GLP-1. The enhancement of the action of GLP-1 receptors using GLP-1 receptor agonists has a beneficial effect on the treatment of diabetes based on the lowering of serum glucose (**Figure 9**). These positive effects on glucose homeostasis coupled with the achievement of weight loss manage to reduce hepatic inflammation and steatosis and to improve liver function tests. The treatment of patients with diabetes melitus type 2 with either exenatide, liraglutide, or semaglutide has proved efficient in the improvement of hepatic steatosis, level of aminotransferases, and inflammatory markers. This effect was clearly associated with the levels of HbA1C and body weight loss. In a study

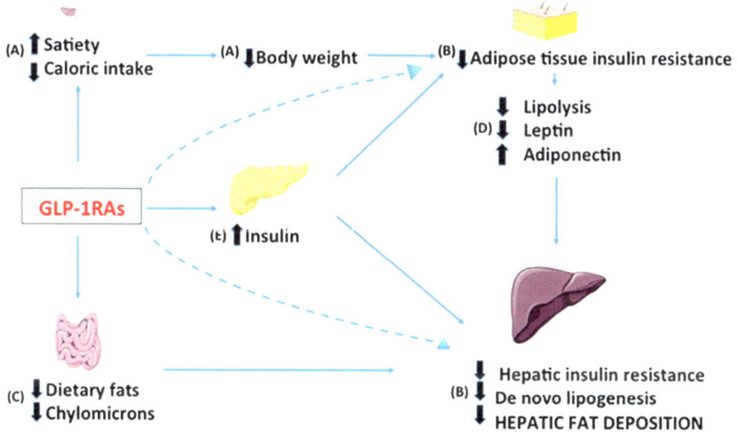

Figure 9.
Action OF GLP-1 agonists In ANFLD/NASH.

including 52 patients with NASH, who received liraglutide or placebo for 48 weeks, a biopsy was performed at the end of treatment in 23 patients receiving liraglutide and 23 patients receiving placebo. Steatosis was improved in nine patients (39%) receiving liraglutide compared to two patients (9%) receiving placebo. These patients were also less likely to present with the progression of fibrosis. Furthermore, compared to the patients that received placebo, the patients with NASH who received semaglutide achieved a greater percentage of resolution of steatosis with no worsening of fibrosis. More studies are underway with the intention to determine the efficacy of these medications in the treatment of NASH with or without cirrhosis [31–33].

The inhibition of DDP-4 has also been a subject of study. DDP-4 inhibitors have shown to reduce hepatic inflammation, fibrosis, and cirrhosis development in animal models. The problem is that the use of sitagliptin did not prove beneficial during the study of the treatment of NAFLD in humans, despite its favorable metabolic effect [34].

3.9 SGLT2 inhibitors

Sodium-glucose cotransporter-2 (SGLT2) inhibitors are a group of sodium-depended glucose transporters which are primarily expressed in the proximal tube epithelium of the kidney and are responsible for the majority (over 90%) of filter glucose reabsorption. Inhibitors of the SGLT2 result in the increased urinary excretion of glucose and the subsequent decrease of serum glucose levels. Their use has been shown to achieve weight loss in many people due to the extensive fluid excretion and the reduction of cardiovascular risk [35].

The above effects have shown that treatment with either Canagliflozin, Empagliflozin, or Dapagliflozine reduced hyperglycemia followed by lower levels of liver enzymes and improvement of liver steatosis. It is hypothesized that the weight loss caused by SGLT2 inhibitors was strongly associated with these effects since SGLT2 is not expressed in the liver (**Figure 10**). A large retrospective study showed a comparative advantage in the use of Canagliflozin and Dapagliflozin in the improvement of hepatic level enzymes independently of body weight loss and HbA1C reduction. More studies with histologic evaluation need to be conducted to evaluate the usefulness of these agents in NAFLD/NASH [36, 37].

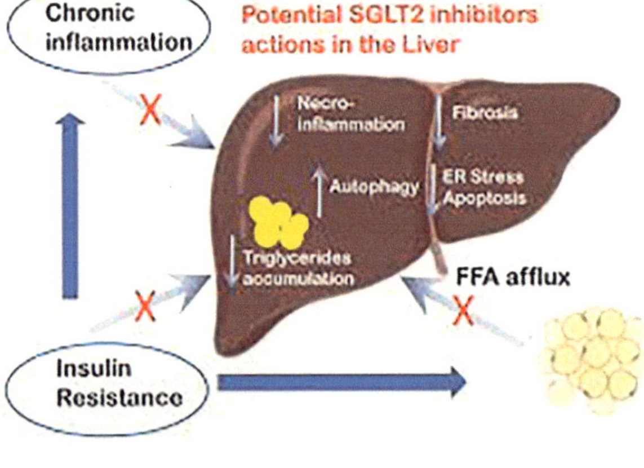

Figure 10.
Potential action of SGLT2 in liver and contribution in NAFLD/NASH treatment.

3.10 Combination treatment

There are currently no randomized clinical trials concerning the combination of treatments mentioned above. From various observation studies, it has been demonstrated that the combination of different treatment methods may have an additional benefit for the patient with NAFLD/NASH compared to individual treatments alone, but further studies should be conducted in that direction. In everyday clinical practice, a combination of different strategies, for example, diet with metformin and statins, is very common, considering that it is the treatment indicated for the conditions which are causally linked to the pathogenesis of NAFLD/NASH.

3.11 Emerging treatments in NAFLD/NASH

Apart from the established treatments, that have been discussed above, there have been also other therapeutic agents that have been shown to be promising in the treatment of NAFLD/NASH (**Figures 11** and **12**). These agents interfere in various stages of the metabolic pathway and may show significant results in improving the radiologic and histologic findings [36].

3.12 Modulation of nuclear transcription factors

Nuclear transcription factors are molecules that bind to their specific ligand and regulate transcription of specific genes and therefore have a beneficial metabolic effect and possibly therapeutic result in the treatment of NAFLD/NASH.

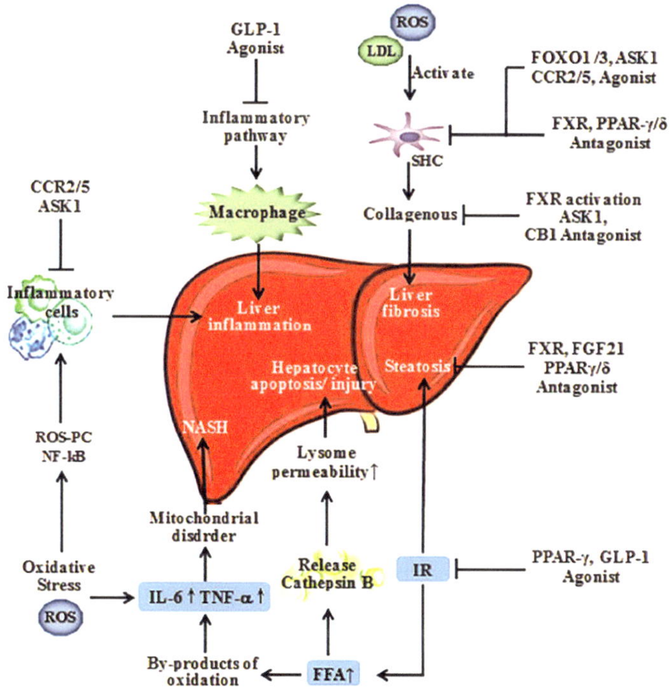

Figure 11.
Metabolic pathways in inflammation in NAFLD/NASH and potential sites of action for new pharmaceutical agents.

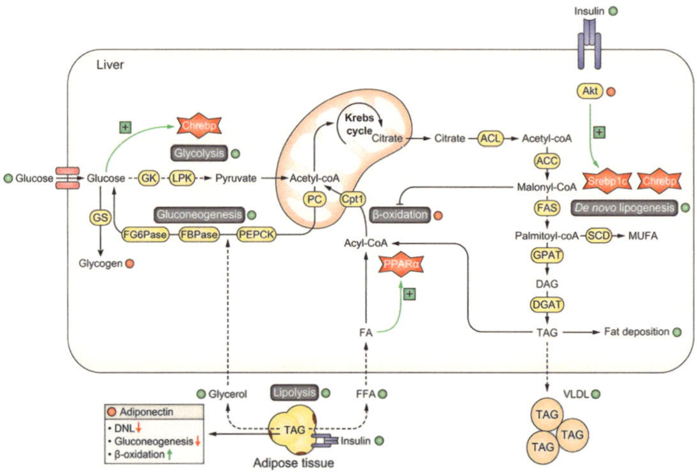

Figure 12.
Metabolic pathways of lipids in NAFLD/NASH and potential sites of action for new pharmaceutical agents.

3.13 Farnesoid X receptor agonist

A crucial regulator of metabolic pathways, including glucose homeostasis, inflammation, and fibrosis, is the farnesoid X receptor (FXR). In patients with NASH, the level of hepatic FXR expression is closely associated with the disease's severity. The liver, kidneys, gut, and adrenal glands all express it. It controls the metabolism of lipoproteins and participates in the production and enterohepatic circulation of bile acids. Bile acid synthesis, hepatic lipogenesis, cholesterol synthesis, and glucose homeostasis are all directly impacted by FXR activation. In animal models, the treatment of FXR agonists has been shown to resolve steatohepatitis and fibrosis as well as prevent the development of NASH. For the treatment of NASH, several synthetic FXR agonists are currently being developed [38].

Bile acids are cholesterol metabolites that are produced in the liver and absorbed from dietary lipids. Type 2 diabetes mellitus raises their levels. In animal models, nor-ursodeoxycholic acid, a synthetic bile acid homolog, has been demonstrated to decrease liver enzymes, fibrosis, and inflammation. Obeticholic acid (OCA), a different modified bile acid, activates the FXR in individuals and raises insulin sensitivity. The FLINT trial, a double-blind placebo, controlled, randomized clinical trial assessed the effectiveness of OCA in patients with NASH without cirrhosis and NAFLD activity score (NAS) > 4 for 72 weeks. Most of these patients had a decrease in the indices of liver fibrosis and inflammation, but they also showed elevated levels of LDL-C, insulin, and a decrease in HDL-C. Because of this, the improvement in liver markers was offset by a worsening of the lipid profile, which required statin therapy. Another ongoing trial (REGENERATE) also demonstrated a slight reduction in fibrosis as compared to placebo, although it did not completely reverse NASH [39].

Tropifexor is another very potent non-bile acid agonist of FXR, which has been shown to be very effective in NASH in animal models and it is under evaluation [40, 41].

3.14 THR-β agonists

THR-a and THR-b are the two isoforms of the nuclear receptor known as the thyroid hormone receptor (THR). The main liver isoform, THR-b, enhances hepatic fatty acid oxidation and lowers steatosis and hyperlipidemia in animal models, whereas THR-a is important in cardiac function. These agonists, e.g., Resmetirom, have been employed in ongoing studies and have demonstrated a favorable impact on NAFLD [42].

3.15 Inhibitors of de novo lipogenesis

3.15.1 ACCs inhibitors

Acetyl-Coa carboxylases (ACCs) promote de novo lipogenesis through the conversion of Acetyl-CoA to Malonyl-CoA, which is a signaling molecule that suppresses fatty acid oxidation. Thus, ACC inhibition reduces lipid accumulation in the liver and stimulates fatty acid oxidation, improving hepatic steatosis and insulin sensitivity in studies in animal models and humans. The problem that arises, is that it also causes hypertriglyceridemia which may further worsen NAFLD [43].

3.15.2 FAS inhibitors

Malonyl-CoA is used by the enzyme fatty acid synthase (FAS) to create saturated long-chain fatty acids. In NAFLD, the enzyme's hepatic expression and activity are botH extremely high, and its suppression results in lower liver lipid levels and improved insulin sensitivity. Therefore, FAS inhibition reduces hepatic steatosis and de novo lipogenesis [44].

3.15.3 SCD-1 inhibitors

Stearoyl-CoA Desaturase-1 (SCD-1) transforms saturated fatty acids into monounsaturated fatty acids and is widely expressed in adipose tissue and the liver. In NAFLD patients, it is quite active. This inhibition leads to reduced steatosis and improvement of insulin sensitivity [42].

3.15.4 DGAT inhibitors

Diacylglycerol acyltransferase (DGAT) catalyzes the esterification of fatty acids. The inhibition of the two isoforms of the enzyme resulted in lower levels of hepatic free acid, glucose, hepatic steatosis, and inflammation [45–47].

3.15.5 Ketohexokinase inhibitors

An enzyme called ketohexokinase encourages the phosphorylation of fructose to fructose-1-phosphate. Fatty acid oxidation enhanced de novo lipogenesis, hepatic steatosis, and inflammation that are brought on by the enzyme's overactivation. Its blockage yields promising outcomes in resolving all the above procedures [46, 47].

3.15.6 MPC inhibitors

The mitochondrial pyruvate carrier (MPC), a combination of two proteins, is crucial for the lipogenesis process in which carbohydrates are converted to fatty acids. Clinical investigations have shown that MPC inhibitors increase insulin sensitivity, reduce liver steatosis, and lower liver enzyme levels.

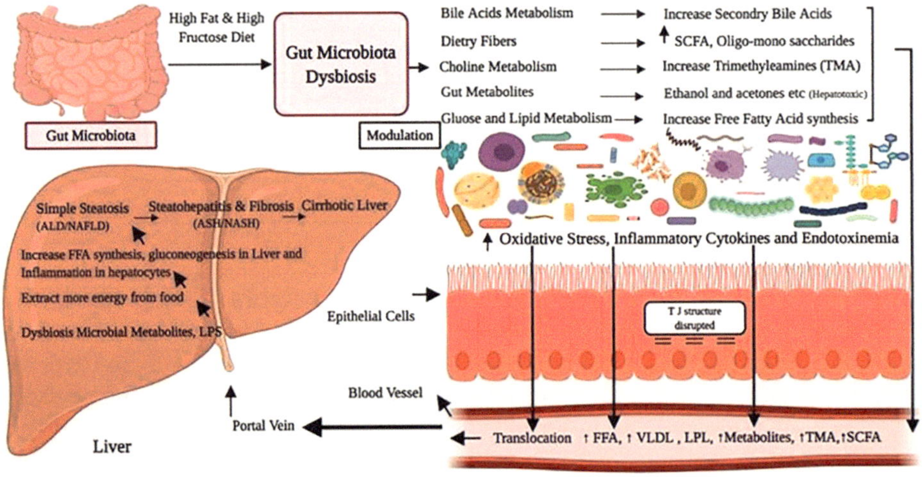

Figure 13.
Gut microbiota and its role in NAFLD/NASH.

3.15.7 FGF (Fibroblast growth factors)

FGF19 is a gastrointestinal hormone that regulates the synthesis of bile acids, the metabolism of glucose, and the oxidation of fatty acids in the liver. FGF19 levels are decreased in NASH patients. Hepatic steatosis and liver enzymes were successfully reduced by the injection of FGF analogs. Another hormone that affects metabolism and energy expenditure is FGF21. Elevated FGF21 levels in NAFLD patients are adversely correlated with reduced insulin sensitivity. High doses of recombinant FGF21 were given to reduce body weight, enhance glucose sensitivity, and change liver and plasma lipid levels [48, 49].

3.15.8 Gut microbiome

The gut microbiome produces substances that are involved in several metabolic pathways and affect the activity of certain metabolites such as bile and fatty acids. Additionally, it is known to play a role in the metabolism of lipids and carbohydrates [50–52]. Numerous studies have demonstrated that the treatment with probiotics, prebiotics, and synbiotics that affect the gut microbiota, may reduce insulin resistance and hepatic inflammation (**Figure 13**). In addition to these, fecal microbiota transplantation (FMT) is being extensively researched and appears to have great promise for the treatment of NAFLD/NASH [51, 53].

4. Conclusions

Nonalcoholic fatty liver disease and its evolution, Non-alcoholic steatohepatitis, constitute a serious cardiometabolic inflammatory process of the liver. Lifestyle modifications such as continued gradual weight loss and exercise are the cornerstone of the therapeutic treatment and have a profound beneficial effect on liver function tests and the co-existing cardiovascular risk. Bariatric surgery could also be advised for certain patients. Several medications have been tried for the treatment of NAFLD/NASH, especially medications that ameliorate the metabolic profile of the patients, insulin sensitivity and lipid oxidation, thus decreasing the lipid burden and improving steatosis and inflammation. Certain new agents have also been under development and show quite promising in the treatment of this complex condition. The implementation of a variety of new agents that target the mechanisms of inflammation and fibrosis in the pathogenesis of NAFLD/NASH will lead us to new effective treatments that will halt the acceleration of the disease and restore normal physiology of the hepatic tissue. Combination therapies may offer a further beneficial effect, but further studies need to be conducted to prove their efficiency.

Conflict of interest

The authors declare no conflict of interest.

Acronyms and abbreviations

BMI	Body Mass Index BMI
SBP	Systolic Blood Pressure
DBP	Diastolic Blood Pressure
CHOL	Cholesterol
LDL-C	LDL-cholesterol
HDL-C	HDL-cholesterol
TGs	triglycerides
HbA1C	glycated hemoglobin
AST	aspartate transaminase
ALT	alanine transaminase
NAFLD	non-alcoholic fatty liver disease
NASH	non-alcoholic steatohepatitis
FIB-4	Mass fibrosis assessment scale.

Author details

Georgios Sfikas[1]* and Ioannis Valsamidis[2]

1 Lipidology and Atherosclerosis Department, General Military Hospital of Thessaloniki, Greece

2 Department of Internal Medicine, General Military Hospital of Thessaloniki, Greece

*Address all correspondence to: geosfik1@gmail.com

References

[1] Ahmed A, Wong RJ, Harrison SA. Nonalcoholic fatty liver disease review: Diagnosis, treatment, and outcomes. Clinical Gastroenterology and Hepatology. 2015;**13**(12):2062-2070

[2] Machado MV, Diehl AM. Pathogenesis of nonalcoholic steatohepatitis. Gastroenterology. 2016;**150**(8):1769-1777

[3] Ekstedt M, Franzén LE, Holmqvist M, Bendtsen P, Mathiesen UL, Bodemar G, et al. Alcohol consumption is associated with progression of hepatic fibrosis in non-alcoholic fatty liver disease. Scandinavian journal of Gastroenterology. 2009;**44**(3):366-374

[4] Adams LA, Anstee QM, Tilg H, Targher G. Non-alcoholic fatty liver disease and its relationship with cardiovascular disease and other extrahepatic diseases. Gut. 2017;**66**(6):1138-1153

[5] Kanwal F, Shubrook JH, Adams LA, Pfotenhauer K, Wong VW, Wright E, et al. Clinical care pathway for the risk stratification and management of patients with nonalcoholic fatty liver disease. Gastroenterology. 2021;**161**(5):1657-1669

[6] Croci I, Coombes JS, Sandbakk SB, Keating SE, Nauman J, Macdonald GA, et al. Non-alcoholic fatty liver disease: Prevalence and all-cause mortality according to sedentary behaviour and cardiorespiratory fitness. The HUNT study. Progress in Cardiovascular Diseases. 2019;**62**(2):127-134

[7] Kim D, Murag S, Cholankeril G, Cheung A, Harrison SA, Younossi ZM, et al. Physical activity, measured objectively, is associated with lower mortality in patients with nonalcoholic fatty liver disease. Clinical Gastroenterology and Hepatology. 2021;**19**(6):1240-1247

[8] Petersen KF, Dufour S, Befroy D, Lehrke M, Hendler RE, Shulman GI. Reversal of nonalcoholic hepatic steatosis, hepatic insulin resistance, and hyperglycemia by moderate weight reduction in patients with type 2 diabetes. Diabetes. 2005;**54**(3):603-608

[9] Promrat K, Kleiner DE, Niemeier HM, Jackvony E, Kearns M, Wands JR, et al. Randomized controlled trial testing the effects of weight loss on nonalcoholic steatohepatitis. Hepatology. 2010;**51**(1):121-129

[10] Chavez-Tapia NC, Tellez-Avila FI, Barrientos-Gutierrez T, Mendez-Sanchez N, Lizardi-Cervera J, Uribe M. Bariatric surgery for non-alcoholic steatohepatitis in obese patients. Cochrane Database of Systematic Reviews. 2010;**1**:5-6

[11] Musso G, Cassader M, Rosina F, Gambino R. Impact of current treatments on liver disease, glucose metabolism and cardiovascular risk in non-alcoholic fatty liver disease (NAFLD): A systematic review and meta-analysis of randomised trials. Diabetologia. 2012;**55**(4):885-904

[12] Chalasani N, Younossi Z, Lavine JE, Charlton M, Cusi K, Rinella M, et al. The diagnosis and management of nonalcoholic fatty liver disease: Practice guidance from the American Association for the Study of Liver Diseases. Hepatology. 2018;**67**(1):328-357

[13] Musso G, Gambino R, Cassader M, Pagano G. A meta-analysis of randomized trials for the treatment of nonalcoholic fatty liver disease. Hepatology. 2010;**52**(1):79-104

[14] Sanyal AJ, Chalasani N, Kowdley KV, McCullough A, Diehl AM, Bass NM, et al. Pioglitazone, vitamin E, or placebo for nonalcoholic steatohepatitis. New England Journal of Medicine. 2010;**362**(18):1675-1685

[15] Hoofnagle JH, Van Natta ML, Kleiner DE, Clark JM, Kowdley KV, Loomba R, et al. Non-alcoholic steatohepatitis clinical research network (NASH CRN). Vitamin E and changes in serum alanine aminotransferase levels in patients with non-alcoholic steatohepatitis. Alimentary Pharmacology & Therapeutics. 2013;**38**(2):134-143

[16] Simon TG, Henson J, Osganian S, Masia R, Chan AT, Chung RT, et al. Daily aspirin use associated with reduced risk for fibrosis progression in patients with nonalcoholic fatty liver disease. Clinical Gastroenterology and Hepatology. 2019;**17**(13):2776-2784

[17] Jiang ZG, Feldbrügge L, Tapper EB, Popov Y, Ghaziani T, Afdhal N, et al. Aspirin use is associated with lower indices of liver fibrosis among adults in the United States. Alimentary Pharmacology & Therapeutics. 2016;**43**(6):734-743

[18] Dongiovanni P, Petta S, Mannisto V, Mancina RM, Pipitone R, Karja V, et al. Statin use and non-alcoholic steatohepatitis in at risk individuals. Journal of Hepatology. 2015;**63**(3):705-712

[19] Athyros V, Tziomalos K, Katsiki N, Gossios T, et al. The impact of smoking on cardiovascular outcomes and comorbidities in statin-treated patients with coronary artery disease: A post hoc analysis of the GREACE study. Current Vascular Pharmacology. 2013;**11**(5):779-784

[20] Pedersen TR, Faergeman O, Kastelein JJ, Olsson AG, Tikkanen MJ, Holme I, et al. High-dose atorvastatin vs usual-dose simvastatin for secondary prevention after myocardial infarction: The IDEAL study: A randomized controlled trial. JAMA. 2005;**294**(19):2437-2445. DOI: 10.1001/jama.294.19.2437

[21] Athyros G et al. Assessing the treatment effect in metabolic syndrome without perceptible diabetes (ATTEMPT): A prospective-randomized study in middle aged men and women. Current Vascular Pharmacology. 2011;**9**(6):647-657

[22] Athyros VG, Giouleme O, Ganotakis ES, Elisaf M, Tziomalos K, Vassiliadis T, et al. Safety and impact on cardiovascular events of long-term multifactorial treatment in patients with metabolic syndrome and abnormal liver function tests: A post hoc analysis of the randomised ATTEMPT study. Archives of Medical Science. 2011;7(5):796-805

[23] Sfikas G, Psallas M, Koumaras C, Imprialos K, Perdikakis E, Doumas M, et al. Prevalence, diagnosis, and treatment with 3 different statins of non-alcoholic fatty liver disease/non-alcoholic steatohepatitis in military personnel. Do genetics play a role? Current Vascular Pharmacology. 2021;**19**(5):572-581

[24] Parker HM, Johnson NA, Burdon CA, Cohn JS, O'Connor HT, George J. Omega-3 supplementation and non-alcoholic fatty liver disease: A systematic review and meta-analysis. Journal of Hepatology. 2012;**56**(4):944-951

[25] Masterton GS, Plevris JN, Hayes PC. Omega-3 fatty acids–a promising novel therapy for non-alcoholic fatty liver disease. Alimentary Pharmacology & Therapeutics. 2010;**31**(7):679-692

[26] Mazza A, Fruci B, Garinis GA, Giuliano S, Malaguarnera R, Belfiore A. The role of metformin in the management of NAFLD. Experimental in Diabetes Research. 2012;**2012**:716

[27] Li Y, Liu L, Wang B, Wang J, Chen D. Metformin in non-alcoholic fatty liver disease: A systematic review and meta-analysis. Biomedical Reports. 2013;**1**(1):57-64

[28] Ratziu V, Giral P, Jacqueminet S, Charlotte F, Hartemann-Heurtier A, Serfaty L, et al. Rosiglitazone for nonalcoholic steatohepatitis: One-year results of the randomized placebo-controlled fatty liver improvement with rosiglitazone therapy (FLIRT) trial. Gastroenterology. 2008;**135**(1):100-110

[29] Promrat K, Lutchman G, Uwaifo GI, Freedman RJ, Soza A, Heller T, et al. A pilot study of pioglitazone treatment for nonalcoholic steatohepatitis. Hepatology. 2004;**39**(1):188-196

[30] Belfort R, Harrison SA, Brown K, Darland C, Finch J, Hardies J, et al. A placebo-controlled trial of pioglitazone in subjects with nonalcoholic steatohepatitis. The New England Journal of Medicine. 2006;**355**(22):2297-2307. DOI: 10.1056/NEJMoa060326

[31] Cusi K, Orsak B, Bril F, Lomonaco R, Hecht J, Ortiz-Lopez C, et al. Long-term pioglitazone treatment for patients with nonalcoholic steatohepatitis and prediabetes or type 2 diabetes mellitus: A randomized trial. Annals of Internal Medicine. 2016;**165**(5):305-315

[32] Ratziu V et al. Elafibranor, an agonist of the peroxisome proliferator− activated receptor− α and− δ, induces resolution of nonalcoholic steatohepatitis without fibrosis worsening. Gastroenterology. 2016;**150**(5):1147-1159

[33] Van Meeteren W, Menso J, Drenth JPH, Tjwa ETTL. Elafibranor: A potential drug for the treatment of nonalcoholic steatohepatitis (NASH). Expert Opinion on Investigational Drugs. 2020;**29**(2):117-123

[34] Armstrong MJ, Gaunt P, Aithal GP, Barton D, Hull D, Parker R, et al. Liraglutide safety and efficacy in patients with non-alcoholic steatohepatitis (LEAN): A multicentre, double-blind, randomised, placebo-controlled phase 2 study. The Lancet. 2016;**387**(10019):679-690

[35] Cusi K. Incretin-based therapies for the Management of Nonalcoholic Fatty Liver Disease in patients with type 2 diabetes. Hepatology. 2019;**69**(6):2318-2322

[36] Newsome PN, Buchholtz K, Cusi K, Linder M, Okanoue T, Ratziu V, et al. NN9931-4296 investigators. A placebo-controlled trial of subcutaneous Semaglutide in nonalcoholic steatohepatitis. The New England Journal of Medicine. 2021;**384**(12):1113-1124

[37] Ideta T, Shirakami Y, Miyazaki T, Kochi T, Sakai H, Moriwaki H, et al. The dipeptidyl peptidase-4 inhibitor teneligliptin attenuates hepatic lipogenesis via AMPK activation in non-alcoholic fatty liver disease model mice. International Journal of Molecular Sciences. 2015;**16**(12):29207-29218

[38] Scheen AJ. Beneficial effects of SGLT2 inhibitors on fatty liver in type 2 diabetes: A common comorbidity associated with severe complications. Diabetes & Metabolism. 2019;**45**(3):213-223

[39] Sumida Y, Yoneda M. Current and future pharmacological therapies for NAFLD/NASH. Journal of Gastroenterology. 2018;**53**(3):362-376

[40] Akuta N, Kawamura Y, Fujiyama S, Sezaki H, Hosaka T, Kobayashi M, et al. SGLT2 inhibitor treatment outcome in nonalcoholic fatty liver disease complicated with diabetes mellitus: The long-term effects on clinical features and liver histopathology. Internal Medicine. 2020;**59**(16):1931-1937

[41] Venetsanaki V, Karabouta Z, Polyzos SA. Farnesoid X nuclear receptor agonists for the treatment of nonalcoholic steatohepatitis. European Journal of Pharmacology. 2019;**863**:172661

[42] Discovery of Tropifexor (LJN452). A highly potent non-bile acid FXR agonist for the treatment of cholestatic liver diseases and nonalcoholic steatohepatitis (NASH). Journal of Medicinal Chemistry. 2017;**60**(24):9960-9973

[43] Ali AH, Carey EJ, Lindor KD. Recent advances in the development of farnesoid X receptor agonists. Annals of Translational Medicine. 2015;**3**(1):5

[44] Arab JP, Karpen SJ, Dawson PA, Arrese M, Trauner M. Bile acids and nonalcoholic fatty liver disease: Molecular insights and therapeutic perspectives. Hepatology (Baltimore, MD). 2017;**65**(1):350-362. DOI: 10.1002/hep.28709

[45] Li X et al. Significant Improvement of NAFLD Activity Scores and Liver Fibrosis by ASC41, a Selective THR-β Agonist, in High Fat Diet Induced NASH SD Rats. Netherlands: Elsevier; 2021

[46] Stiede K, Miao W, Blanchette HS, Beysen C, Harriman G, Harwood HJ Jr, et al. Acetyl-coenzyme A carboxylase inhibition reduces de novo lipogenesis in overweight male subjects: A randomized, double-blind, crossover study. Hepatology. 2017;**66**(2):324-334

[47] Aljohani AM, Syed DN, Ntambi JM. Insights into stearoyl-CoA desaturase-1 regulation of systemic metabolism. Trends in Endocrinology and Metabolism. 2017;**28**:831-842

[48] Kotronen A, Seppänen-Laakso T, Westerbacka J, Kiviluoto T, Arola J, Ruskeepaa AL, et al. Hepatic stearoyl-CoA desaturase (SCD)-1 activity and diacylglycerol but not ceramide concentrations are increased in the nonalcoholic human fatty liver. Diabetes. 2009;**58**(1):203-208

[49] Degirolamo C, Sabbà C, Moschetta A. Therapeutic potential of the endocrine fibroblast growth factors FGF19, FGF21 and FGF23. Nature Reviews Drug Discovery. 2016;**15**(1):51-69

[50] Yamaguchi K, Yang L, McCall S, Huang J, Yu XX, Pandey SK, et al. Inhibiting triglyceride synthesis improves hepatic steatosis but exacerbates liver damage and fibrosis in obese mice with nonalcoholic steatohepatitis. Hepatology. 2007;**45**(6):1366-1374

[51] Saxena A, Chidsey K, Somayaji V, Ogden A, Duvvuri S. Diacylglycerol acyltransferase 2 (DGAT2) inhibitor PF-06865571 reduces liver fat by MRI-PDFF after 2 weeks in adults with NAFLD. Hoboken, NJ: Wiley;

[52] Leung C, Rivera L, Furness JB, Angus PW. The role of the gut microbiota in NAFLD. Nature Reviews Gastroenterology & Hepatology. 2016;**13**(7):412-425

[53] Safari Z, Gérard P. The links between the gut microbiome and non-alcoholic fatty liver disease (NAFLD). Cellular and Molecular Life Sciences. 2019;**76**(8):1541-1558